Eat Yourself Fit

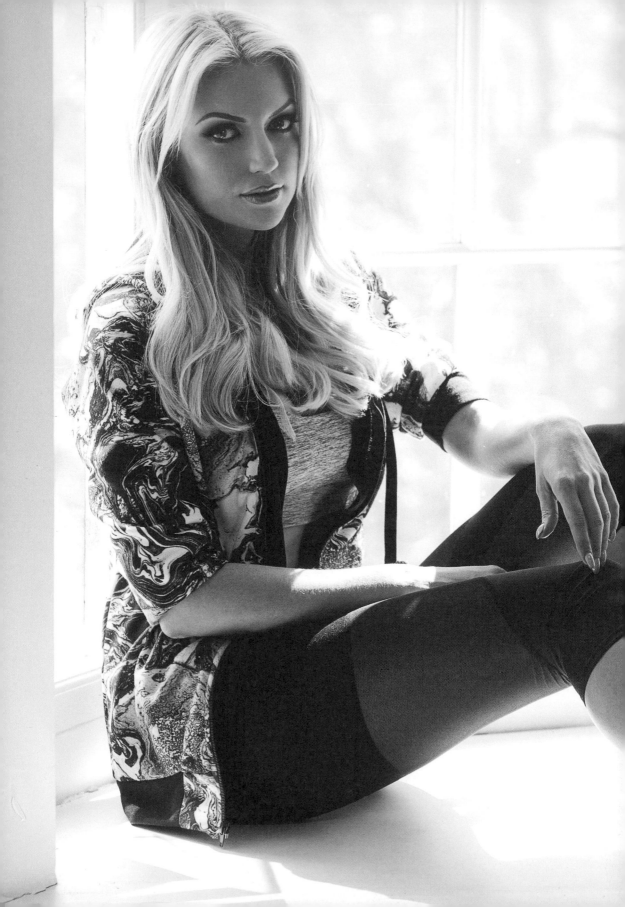

EAT YOURSELF FIT

ROSANNA DAVISON

GILL BOOKS

Gill Books
Hume Avenue
Park West
Dublin 12
www.gillbooks.ie

Gill Books is an imprint of M.H. Gill & Co.

© Rosanna Davison 2016

978 07171 7155 2

Designed by www.grahamthew.com
Food photography by Neil Hurley
Lifestyle photography by Gavin Glave
Food and props styled by Jette Virdi
Photography location courtesy of Mags Clark-Smith magsclarksmith.com
Edited by Kristin Jensen
Indexed by Eileen O'Neill
Printed by BZ Graf, Poland

PROPS
Article: www.articledublin.com
Industry & Co: www.industryandco.com
Scout: scoutdublin.com

This book is typeset in Perpetua 11pt on 14 pt

A CIP catalogue record for this book is available from the British Library.

5 4 3 2 1

ACKNOWLEDGEMENTS

Thank you to the brilliant team at Gill Books for
your constant support and belief in me, and for
giving me the chance to write my second book.

To my amazing family, I am grateful beyond words
for your love, encouragement and advice.

Thank you most of all to my wonderful husband, Wes,
for your unwavering support, patience and love, and for
taking your job as chief recipe tester very seriously indeed.

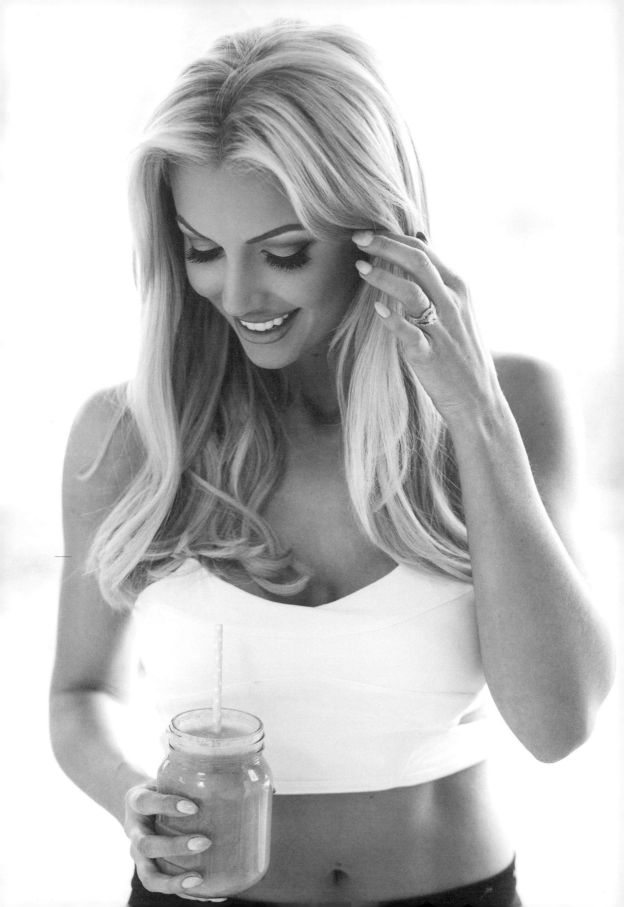

CONTENTS

BACK TO BASICS

"Take care of your body.
It's the only place you have to live."

JIM ROHN

Eat Yourself Fit combines good food, easy-to-follow recipes and functional nutrition with fitness information and practical tips to help with stress management and emotional well-being. I have focused on bringing together body and mind in a unique holistic approach to create a sustainable and health-promoting lifestyle.

We live in a busy, stressful and often demanding world in which our own health and wellness needs can be pushed down the list of priorities to make room for family, friends, work, study and life. Many of us need to find a way to re-establish that elusive balance between mind, body and spirit and to discover a way to take better charge of our own physical and emotional needs by listening to the signs our bodies share with us and becoming more tuned in to them.

It may take some time to really learn about how your body works once you start paying attention to its subtle signals. I'm a strong advocate of following the lifestyle that suits you best because we're all biochemically unique individuals. Yet there is a powerful interconnection between body and mind in all of us and I firmly believe that full health, wellness and contentment within ourselves is best achieved by taking the time to nourish both.

In this book, I have created a food for fitness plan that will help achieve real results. You will get more from the food you eat, helping to boost your energy levels, reduce body fat, improve muscle tone, lift your mood, manage stress and even enhance the quality of your sleep.

I explain all you need to know about the most effective foods and exercises for maximising your workouts, sculpting your body and ensuring that you feel strong, fit, healthy and confident.

Packed with information on health and fitness, recipes and my favourite tips and secrets, this book has everything you need to help you reach your health and fitness potential, whatever your own personal goals may be.

I hope you enjoy reading my story, trying out my fitness tips and food plan and tasting the wide range of delicious recipes as much as I have loved sharing them with you.

In fitness and health,

Rosanna x

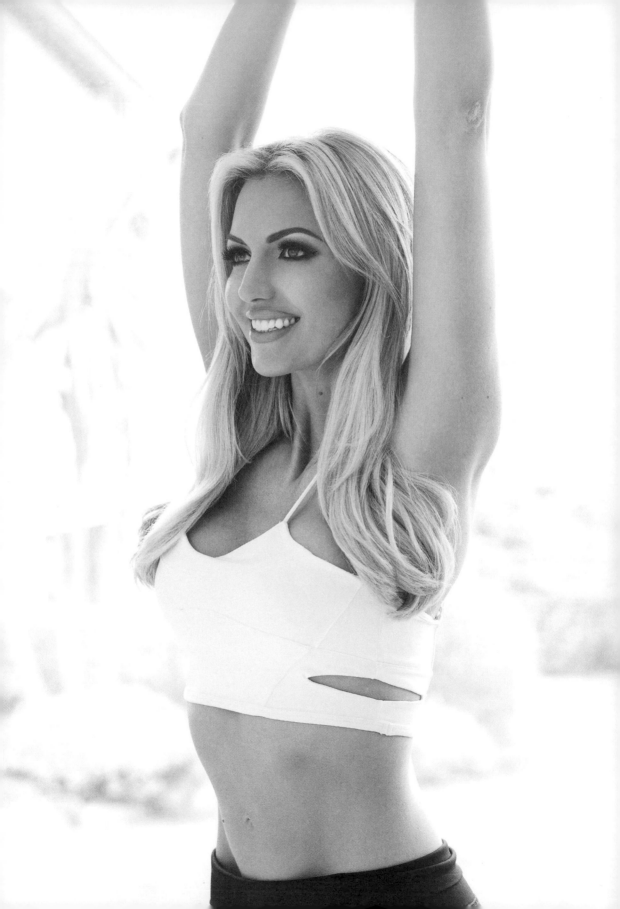

PART I

MY FITNESS STORY

"Living a healthy lifestyle will
only deprive you of poor health,
lethargy and fat."

JILL JOHNSON

I have always loved sports and fitness. As a pony-mad little girl, I dreamed of being a professional show jumper, representing my country on a feisty chestnut mare. At 11 years old, I was building fences in the garden with bamboo poles and jumping the family black Labrador over a pretend show jumping course while dressed in my jodhpurs, boots and riding hat. It was quite a sight. I went on to own a pony for five years and I enjoyed riding her in many gymkhanas and show jumping competitions.

This led to a love for hurdles and high jumping, so I joined an athletics club at the age of 15 and competed for my school and club at both Leinster and all-Ireland levels, bringing home enough hard-earned medals to just about satisfy my bouncy competitive streak.

Throughout my primary and secondary school years, I held a place on the hockey, netball and cricket teams between taking tennis lessons and even badminton too.

At the age of 18, I took up Pilates in a new studio close to my family home. It wasn't long before I sat my Leaving Certificate exams, and I found that the twice-weekly classes really helped to give me the focus and mental clarity I needed amongst the chaos and stress of exam prep. It was a different type of fitness than I had been used to, much more slow and controlled, with a focus on core strength, posture, developing long and lean muscles, mindfulness and body awareness. That started my long-term love of Pilates and it still plays an important role in my fitness regime.

With all the running I did for hockey, netball and athletics training after school and the matches every weekend, I never even had to think about my weight or what I was eating. In fact, we would refuel after a hockey game with copious quantities of digestive biscuits and sugary lemonade. I was on the slightly lanky side as a teenager, all awkward coltish limbs, a self-conscious lopsided smile and plenty of zits.

It was only when I began my first year at university in Dublin that I began putting on weight and I really noticed my body shape changing. In that first year, like many of my peers, I was spending too many afternoons and evenings downing sugary blue alcopops in the student bar, then soaking it all up with chips and crisps. I wasn't exercising to nearly the same degree as I did during school, and with my newfound freedom, student night-clubs and bars had replaced the hockey pitch.

Looking back, I was a serious sugar addict. Early lectures were eased with a sugary cappuccino in hand, I reached for a processed cereal bar for the mid-morning munchies and sweetened yogurts were a frequent afternoon snack. I had even been known to guzzle syrupy, caffeinated energy drinks to power me through exams.

By the end of my first year in college, I had managed to return to my normal weight, partly from joining the college gym and partly from a girly holiday to Greece in which we endeavoured to exist on €5 a day. This meant that more money was spent on cheap ouzo than nourishing food. Definitely not to be recommended, but a lot of fun for a 19-year-old student with very few responsibilities.

Later that summer, I was thrown headfirst and without much warning into the glossy, glittering world of beauty pageants when I won Miss Ireland in August 2003. This led to me winning Miss World 2003 in China that December. The Miss World Organisation stipulated that my weight (and hair colour) must remain the same throughout the year.

For a young woman in a whole new industry, that felt like a lot of pressure. I became much more aware of my diet, fitness and lifestyle habits. At that stage, I had figured out that I had more energy and generally felt better by eating a vegetarian diet. Plus choosing veggies, salads and soups over heavier animal-based foods when I was home and eating out meant that I was finding it easier to maintain my weight, my energy levels improved and my immune system strengthened too. Gone were the frequent niggling coughs and sore throats, and I had all the energy I needed for the often gruelling long-haul trips to China for a weekend of Miss World charity events.

Of course, that was just my personal experience and not everybody will react in the same way to a change in diet and lifestyle. This book is by no means about trying to turn you into a vegetarian. Rather, it is designed to encourage more of an awareness of the relationship between nutrition, body fat and fitness, your mood, emotions and even your sleep. As I will explain in the following chapters, this book is about fitting together the pieces of the puzzle and the various elements that lead to a balanced, healthy and happy lifestyle, and increased body confidence too.

My weight remained pretty stable throughout my early twenties, bar the usual slight hormonal fluctuations. I maintained a balanced diet and stayed active, running regularly in charity events. I completed my first half marathon in under two hours.

At that point, I was 27 and had recently started eating a fully plant-based diet, intended as a week-long experiment in my college nutrition course, so that I would be able to explain the pros and cons to future clients. For six to eight months prior to that, I had been focusing on weight training and had been going to a personal trainer a few times a week for intense sessions. I loved how weight training made me feel strong and was really starting to sculpt my body, helping to lower body fat and increase muscle tone. I had put myself on a high-protein, low-carb 'training diet' because I thought it was the best way to build lean muscle and make the most of my workouts. This meant that plenty of whey protein shakes, egg whites and fat-free cottage cheese made up the bulk of my diet.

And you know what? I was feeling awful and getting progressively more lethargic, tired and reliant on caffeine. I simply could not understand how my new 'healthy' diet was making me feel so listless.

Having dreaded trying out the plant-based diet because I expected it to be difficult and dull, by the end of the week I felt better than I had in a long time. In fact, the difference was dramatic. The extra fibre had initially been a bit of a shock to my digestive system and I had felt very bloated for the first few days, but once that had settled down, I began to feel full of energy and enthusiasm. I even started sleeping better too. I decided to keep up the same style of eating for another week, and again enjoyed even more improvements to my energy levels. Even my skin was starting to look brighter and fresher, and I found that I was far less reliant on coffee to kick start my day.

To my amazement, by the end of the third week, my normal clothes were starting to hang loose on me. I had dropped a dress size in those first few weeks without even intending to. The new eating plan had been about trying something different and feeling better doing it, and I hadn't once thought about my calorie intake. I was eating even more food than usual, but it was all high-fibre plant food with plenty of legumes, leafy greens and some healthy fats like avocado, nuts and seeds too. I was munching on huge kale salads, sweet potato, quinoa, lentils, chickpeas, green smoothies and berries.

Doing the supermarket shop was a new and daunting experience, but I soon found that I could get pretty much everything I needed in my local supermarket, and much of it was cheaper than my previous way of eating. I found that weekly farmers' markets were a super place to stock up on loads of fruit and veggies, and I also invested in a Vitamix blender to whip up my soups, dips, smoothies and my new addiction, frozen banana 'ice cream'.

The next happy surprise came a couple of months into eating a plant-based diet, when I realised that my fitness and endurance levels were noticeably improving. I was able to run faster and for longer. On top of that, I noticed my body composition changing, as I was reducing body fat and increasing muscle tone. I was diligent about drinking a daily green smoothie, filled with Popeye's favourite muscle-building spinach, and even now, my signature green goddess smoothie (page 133) is a key part of my health and fitness regime.

For the following few years, I happily enjoyed all the benefits of my plant-based diet and it became second nature. Colds, sniffles, coughs and flus became a thing of the past. I gleefully powered through the winter months without so much as a runny nose, while so many others around me took days off work sick.

However, my next weight and health wobble came during the summer of 2014. Wes and I got married in a beautiful ceremony in Ibiza in early June 2014, following weeks of a healthy eating and fitness regime to prepare for the big day and to feel as confident as possible in my wedding gown. Sugar and alcohol were off limits and I spent hours in the gym toning up. There's nothing like a wedding to boost your motivation.

But weddings also come with plenty of opportunities to indulge in wine and Champagne. I rarely drink wine as the yeast doesn't agree with me, but I let myself off the hook and enjoyed wine with dinner over the course of our stay in Ibiza. We took off on honeymoon to the Seychelles the following week and we fully indulged in a pre-dinner cocktail, wine with our meal and three large buffet meals a day.

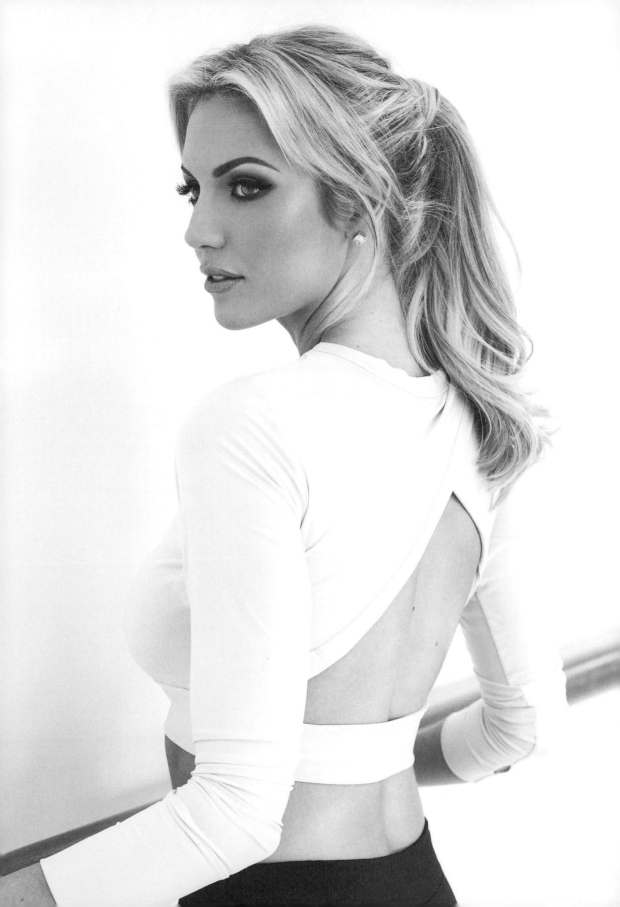

I arrived home glowing with newlywed bliss, but carrying at least an extra stone of weight. And then panic struck. My clothes had been getting progressively tighter on our honeymoon, to the point where I couldn't wear certain outfits, but I had brushed that off as a bit of extra water weight from the humidity. Yet when that 'water weight' still hadn't budged from my tummy, hips, bottom and thighs a few weeks after we got home and I had to buy jeans in a bigger size, I knew I had to take more intense measures.

Body size is a highly sensitive and very personal issue, and I'm well aware that there are plenty of women and men who would like to bulk up and develop some extra curves. We come in all different shapes and sizes, and that diversity is something to be celebrated. But it's also important to feel comfortable and confident in your own skin, and having been lean for most of my life, I simply wasn't feeling good about myself.

Determined to get my confidence back and feel like myself again, I put myself on a strict calorie-controlled eating plan for two months. Overall, I aimed to bulk up my diet with loads of vegetables and smaller amounts of healthy fats, beans and legumes and grains like quinoa, oats and millet.

This was not a 'diet'. I'm not a fan of quick fixes, and I firmly believe that the diet industry is set up to keep the consumer coming back time and time again in a frustrating cycle of fat loss and gain. Most diets are not sustainable or practical as a lifestyle, and dieters often end up piling any lost weight back on when they begin to eat normally again. Humans are not built to be able to override feelings of hunger, and a high-calorie binge often follows a period of drastically cutting back on food. It's not because you're weak or greedy – it's an inbuilt biological need to sustain your brain and major organs with food. Food is needed to keep you *alive*. It's not something to be feared or feel guilty about enjoying.

I took a sustainable lifestyle approach to weight loss, never going hungry, exercising regularly and allowing myself a treat now and then if I really fancied it. Through the food and exercise plan I designed for myself I managed to lose the weight I had gained.

Unfortunately, there are no magic bullets to fitness and patience really is key. It was hugely challenging at times and I found myself turning down invitations to parties and events just so I wouldn't be tempted by treats. Motivation is a big part of working towards a healthier lifestyle, but perfection is not what it's about either, as temptations will always arise. Instead, it's about moving in the right direction and learning how to make more positive choices.

I'm generally not interested in calorie counting, as it's not that practical for anyone leading a busy lifestyle or who has to eat out frequently. Instead, I'm a firm advocate of helping people to understand portion sizes and to choose nutrient-dense foods over calorie-dense foods. This is a more sustainable way of enjoying your food without becoming obsessed with logging every morsel eaten. However, if you're serious about weight loss, then calories do naturally become a part of it, especially the quality of the calories consumed. Eating nutrient-dense food in every mouthful becomes even more important because your body needs certain nutrients every day to function normally and for you to feel your best.

My weight stays pretty much stable now and I'm back to feeling fit, energetic, healthy and strong. My journey to fitness, health and really understanding my body has been long and filled with bumps along the way, but with every mistake I made, I learned a valuable lesson — and I'm still learning.

My focus has never been about looking skinny or fitting into the tiniest jeans size possible, and I don't believe that it should be for anybody. I have struggled over the years to find the right balance for my body, and I finally feel that I've managed to figure out the food and fitness regime that works for me, and will hopefully work for you too.

This is not a diet book. I wrote it to inspire, inform and give you an insight into my own wellness journey and to share my tried-and-tested tips, fitness secrets and favourite recipes for helping you to become your healthiest, strongest, fittest, happiest and most energetic self. Strong really is the new skinny, and it's definitely here to stay.

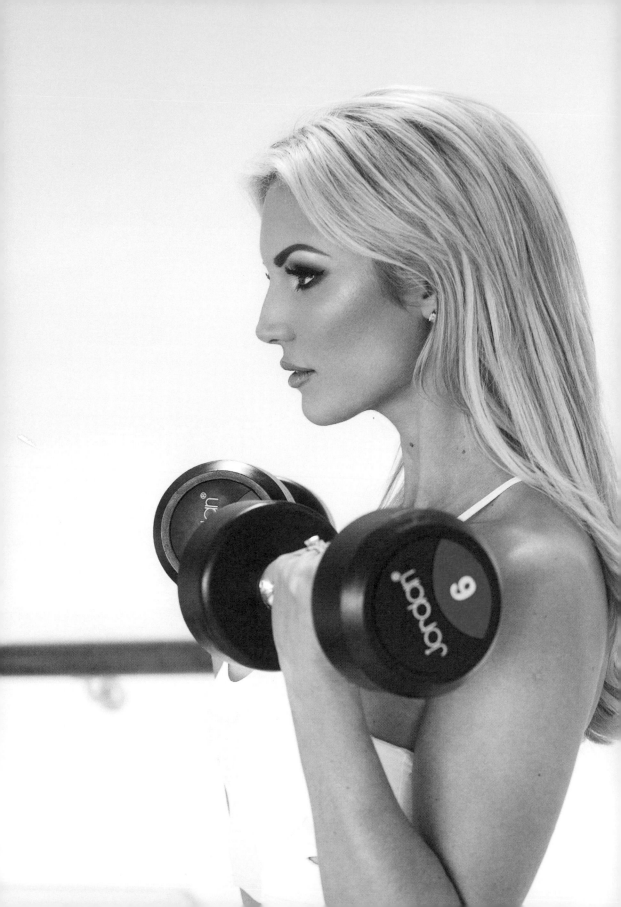

PART 2

FIT FOR LIFE

"Those who think they have no time
for bodily exercise will sooner or later
have to find time for illness."

EDWARD STANLEY

Nutritious food and fitness are a match made in heaven, and like any great relationship, they bring out each other's very best qualities. The closest thing to a magic bullet for slowing down the ageing process and developing a healthy, strong, fit and lean physique is that golden combination of good nutrition and exercise.

Your entire physical and emotional well-being benefits enormously from this dynamic duo. Increasing your heart rate and working up a sweat regularly through exercise boosts digestion and elimination, blood flow and lymphatic drainage, enhances your fitness and energy levels, supports fat burning, reduces cholesterol levels, improves insulin sensitivity and may even combat feelings of anxiety and depression while boosting your mood with feel-good endorphins.

The scientific consensus supports regular exercise, and suggests that 'moderate fitness' can be achieved in as few as 10 weeks by daily walking, cycling and even tending to the garden. In fact, exercise and the path to fitness can incorporate a whole range of movements and different ways to increase your heart rate and work up a sweat.

We all have to start somewhere

For the majority of people, the most daunting and intimidating part of getting fit is where to begin. It can feel like we're constantly bombarded with conflicting information about health, fat loss and fitness, making it almost impossible to know what to start with.

There seems to be a vast array of diet plans, powders, tablets, shakes, bars, websites, blogs, gyms and fitness experts trying to sell us their products, which is why it is so important to separate fact from marketing. Confusing the public can work in favour of the companies pushing their wares, as it may encourage us to blindly buy into their trends.

Just like food and nutrition, fitness works best when it's kept as simple as possible. Different types of exercise work for different people, and discovering what you like most is the key to viewing exercise as enjoyable and getting the very most out of it. It should be fun, challenging and changed up regularly to make sure it never gets boring.

Do you love to dance? Unwind in a yoga class? Or maybe jogging along a scenic coastal route really helps to uplift and energise you? No matter how disciplined and determined you may be, it's very difficult to motivate yourself to get active when it's something you don't enjoy.

I used to love running until my hip began to hurt after long-distance runs. I pushed myself for a while longer and forced myself out for runs, until one day I just stopped completely because I was beginning to really dislike running. You can always swap one type of regime for another that suits your age and body type better, and now I much prefer the cross-trainer or bicycle for my cardiovascular exercise.

I have also found that in my thirties, I'm more interested in doing slower and more controlled exercises that really build my core strength and muscle groups, such as Pilates and resistance training in the gym. I used to love boxing and high-intensity treadmill sprints in my twenties, but they don't suit me so much anymore.

Another important part of staying fit and active is making sure it slots into your lifestyle and that you're not compromising your health or sleep. If you're dragging yourself out of bed at 5am to hit the treadmill before work, there's probably only so long you can keep it up before illness or injury prevents you. A bad experience can quite easily lead to a loss of confidence in your own abilities and even cause you to resent exercise.

If you have joined a gym or fitness class and aren't sure where to begin, then don't be afraid to ask questions and look for help. Most good gyms will have fitness experts on hand to advise you. It's so important to do certain exercises properly to avoid injury, and weightlifting in particular can become more risky if you're not protecting your neck and back.

Want to change your body shape?

The number of times a week you train will depend on your own lifestyle and personal goals. To maintain your current body, aim to work out three times a week. To really change or sculpt your body, increase it to four to six times a week. You certainly don't need to spend two hours in the gym each time. Step up the intensity, taking as few rests as possible, and you can get a very good workout done in 30–40 minutes.

My top tip for building muscle tone and really changing your body shape by reducing body fat and increasing lean muscle is to work the muscle until the point of failure. You can do this with heavier weights for three or four sets of 10–12 reps, or lighter weights for more sets and reps. To find out which approach suits you, I recommend that you meet with a trainer before beginning a new exercise regimen. Good technique is crucial if you are to avoid injury and get the most out of your workouts. Add to this an eating plan to support your hard work in the gym, and the results will soon begin to show.

Try to get into the habit of pushing yourself through those final few reps that you think you can't manage, because they're the ones that really count. Your brain will probably try to tell your body to stop or that it can't go on. But mental strength and determination are key, and overcoming your brain's messages to quit will make all the difference to your fitness and body shape.

To burn body fat, my advice is to do cardiovascular exercise four to five times a week. High-intensity interval training is a tried-and-tested way to torch calories. It can be done on the treadmill, stationary bike, cross-trainer or any other cardio machine. I like to cycle or cross-train for 30 seconds as fast as I possibly can, then slow it right down for 30 seconds and repeat for about 20 minutes. As you get fitter, you can adapt it for a longer sprint time and less recovery time. This type of high-intensity training helps to burn body fat without reducing lean muscle mass, which is also ideal for boosting your metabolism.

Types of exercise

Different types of exercise achieve different health, muscle-toning and cardio-vascular goals. My advice is to combine a variety of movements to achieve a great boost to your endurance, flexibility and strength. The key is to keep it consistent for the best results.

I've tried out many different types of fitness classes and regimes, from aerobics classes to kickboxing and yoga. As much as I enjoyed them, I find that I get the very best overall results from combining weight training with Pilates and cardio.

Do you struggle to make time for regular exercise? I'm often busy working or travelling and finding the time can be difficult, so I have to get inventive with workout routines. It's possible to do a demanding workout in the space of 10–20 minutes at home using your own body weight, training bands or a TRX, and I've been known to sprint up and down hotel staircases to work up a sweat!

The point is to make exercise an enjoyable part of your lifestyle so that it's a fun challenge, it never feels like a chore and you miss it when you don't have a chance to do it.

RESISTANCE TRAINING

Weight or resistance training is incredibly important for strengthening all your muscles, for improving your ratio of lean muscle to fat mass and for sculpting your body.

Like many other women, I used to worry that lifting weights would bulk me up like a bodybuilder, so I lifted tiny weights inconsistently and instead focused on cardiovascular exercise. When I was eventually convinced to try proper weight training, I couldn't believe the difference it made to my body.

It became so much easier to stay slim and toned, as weight training boosts your metabolism by encouraging the body to burn calories for hours after the session while your muscle fibres repair themselves. Of course, I didn't bulk up but actually slimmed down, as a pound of muscle takes up less space than a pound of fat.

Women don't have enough of the hormone testosterone needed to bulk up in the way that men can. Instead, we produce more oestrogen, which makes us prone to storing fat. Weight training is especially beneficial for women, as it encourages your bones to continuously rebuild and strengthen themselves, helping to prevent the onset of osteomalacia and osteoporosis.

It's important to train each major muscle and muscle group in the body at least once a week for visible results. Resistance training tones, tightens and sculpts your body while reducing body fat levels and improving muscle tone. I would encourage everybody to consider adding weightlifting to their fitness regimen.

Exercises such as squats, lunges, press-ups and planks work a number of major muscles and can all be done without equipment, using your body weight in the comfort of your own home. As long as you don't suffer from lower body joint problems, I advise you to incorporate regular squats into your routine. They work your glutes, quads, hamstrings and core and even help to improve your posture, plus they encourage fat burning by boosting your metabolism and increasing the production of growth hormones.

To avoid injury if you're brand new to it, it would be best to start out with a trainer or workout buddy who knows what they're doing. If you're over the age of 35 or have had a sedentary lifestyle for some time, it would be best to arrange a one-on-one consultation with a health and fitness expert before beginning an exercise programme.

CARDIOVASCULAR EXERCISE
Cardiovascular or aerobic exercise boosts your body's ability to burn oxygen and glucose while benefitting your cardio-vascular system by increasing the blood flow to your heart, lungs and muscles and carrying oxygen via your blood to all your tissues. More oxygen-rich blood in the tiny

capillaries near your skin's surface means plenty of nutrients reach your skin to help keep it looking fresh, radiant and young.

As little as half an hour a day of power walking, jogging, swimming, cycling or dancing helps to keep you lean, builds a stronger heart, and supports your lymphatic system in draining away toxic build-up.

I always aim to do some form of cardio exercise about four to five times a week, whether it's a cycle, a brisk walk or using an exercise machine in the gym such as the cross-trainer, step machine or Wattbike. The impact that it has on my alertness, mood, happiness, health, fitness and body fat makes it time very well spent.

FLEXIBILITY
Depending on the type of class, exercises like Pilates and yoga don't always get your heart pumping in quite the same way as cardiovascular and high-intensity resistance training or circuits, but they strengthen and elongate muscles, help to improve joint health, tighten your core muscles, lengthen your spine, help your posture, oxygenate your blood and body cells and offer countless benefits for emotional well-being and stress management.

I have loved Pilates for years, and I really like how well it balances out the other types of training I do. Most weeks, I will do three to four classes and the routine changes each time. Some will be more focused on breathing and core, while others really challenge all your muscles and give you a sweaty, full-body strength and conditioning workout.

STRETCHING

Stretching before and after a workout can be just as important as the workout itself. It helps to prevent injury, increases blood flow and encourages long, lean muscles and good flexibility.

It also makes a big difference to muscle tightness and pain over the day or two after an intense workout; sometimes this lingering discomfort can put people off continuing their fitness regime. Take a few minutes to warm up and stretch well before a workout, then a few minutes to cool down and stretch afterwards to avoid those muscle cramps and soreness as much as possible.

CORE VALUES

The band of muscles around your mid-section that make up your core, such as your abdominals and obliques, are probably the most important of all to keep strong for overall strength, fitness and protection from injury. Almost every movement you make, from lifting shopping bags out of the boot of your car to pulling out a chair from the kitchen table and lifting weights in the gym, relies on your core muscles.

In nearly every resistance or Pilates workout I do, I'm working and strengthening my core. Whether you're a cardio bunny or a weights devotee, working with a strong core can really help to improve your overall posture and form.

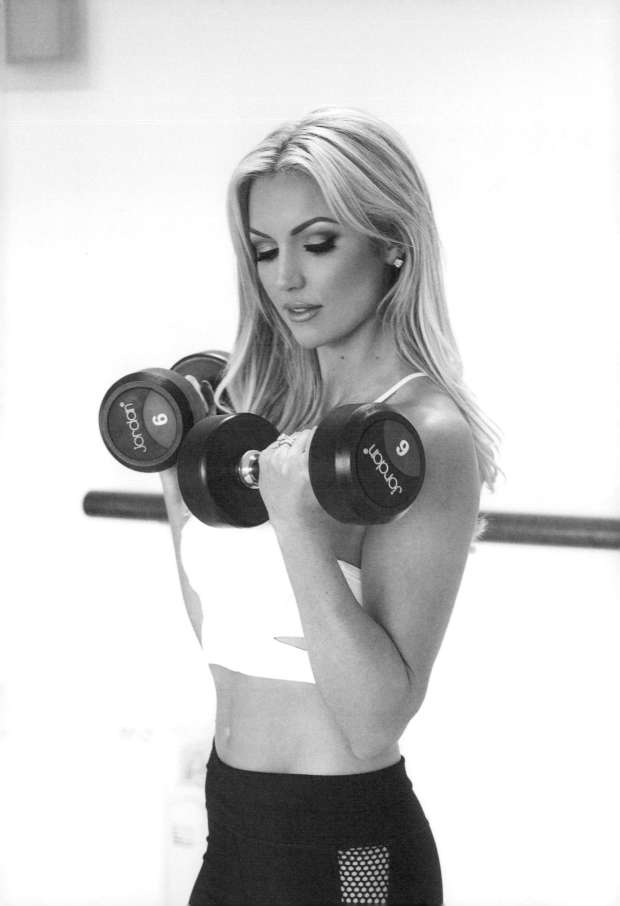

MY POSITIVE FITNESS TIPS

I'm often asked about how I fit regular exercise into my busy routine and to suggest ways for others to manage it in a practical way. We all lead hectic lives packed with work, family and domestic commitments amongst many others, and I fully understand how difficult it can be to squeeze a bit of time into the day to exercise. Getting myself into the gym or outside to exercise is as much of a struggle sometimes as it is for anyone else, believe me. There are some days when I feel really revved up and ready to go, but others when I feel tired and unmotivated. And almost every day, there's something 'more important' to be done first.

But one of my main sources of comfort, support, stability and feel-good factor, other than my husband, friends and family, of course, has been my exercise routine. Yes, it can feel like torture to get yourself to the gym or park, but have you ever regretted a workout? I certainly haven't. Being self-employed and working in an industry where plans can change literally at the last minute, fitness has been a constant and reliable friend to me, always guaranteed to energise my body and brighten my mood. Here are my top five positive fitness tips.

1

VIEW IT AS TIME OUT FOR YOURSELF RATHER THAN A PUNISHMENT

I like to view it as time out from a hectic life. Plus it helps to calm me because I put all of my mental energy into focusing on the exercise I'm doing.

Exercise oxygenates the body and brain, releases happy endorphins and makes you feel strong, healthy and capable enough to take on life's challenges. It's also excellent for your heart and lung health, helps to maintain a healthy weight and to improve insulin sensitivity in a world where many people eat far too much refined sugar.

2

MAKE IT A PART OF YOUR EVERYDAY LIFE

Exercise is as much a part of my daily routine as my breakfast is. It's not something that I have to think about and decide on — I just do it and get on with my day. Removing the decision to exercise because it's as normal a part of your routine as brushing your teeth or showering helps to cancel out the temptation to skip it.

3

BRING YOUR GYM GEAR EVERYWHERE

I keep a pair of old runners in the boot of my car in case I meet up with a friend and we decide to go for a walk instead of sitting down for food or a coffee. Similarly, I take my gym gear on every overnight work trip I do abroad, as it's normal for me to squeeze in a workout between the plane and whatever job I'm doing. If I'm tired from an early flight, a blast in the gym or run in the fresh air works wonders.

4

EAT TO SUPPORT YOUR BODY AND MIND

Good nutrition is crucial to fitness and emotional well-being. I know I couldn't lead a busy life and stay fit and healthy without eating the way that I do, with foods that nourish every cell in my body. Back in my early twenties, when I was a sugar addict and unaware of the connection between food and my body, I used to eat whatever junk I craved and then wonder why I'd get constant colds, sniffles and sore throats. All the recipes in this book are designed to deeply nourish your body and support fitness, health and weight loss goals.

5

TAKE RESPONSIBILITY FOR YOUR ACTIONS

One trait that all fit and motivated people share is discipline. It's easy to make excuses to skip exercise or do a less than high-standard job at anything in life. But taking responsibility for your actions and knowing that nobody else but you is accountable for the consequences has always helped me achieve my goals. Hard work, intelligent effort and avoiding the temptation to blame somebody else when things don't always go right is a key combination to success in fitness and in life.

HOW TO BOOST YOUR MOTIVATION

As much as I love keeping fit, I definitely have days when I'm feeling disinterested. It's only human. But the glowing, virtuous feeling you get afterwards makes it all worthwhile. Just getting yourself outside or to the gym is half the battle. Here are my favourite motivation tips.

1

TRICK YOURSELF

I love this tip and it pretty much works every time. If I'm not feeling very energetic, I'll go to the gym and tell myself that I'll do a light and easy 10 minutes on the bike or cross-trainer, nothing too strenuous. Then if I still don't feel like it, I'll go home and have a much-improved resolve the following day. And guess what? Nine times out of ten, I'll feel so much more energised and raring to go after that light warm-up that I'll stay on to do a proper workout and feel great afterwards.

2

PUMP UP THE MUSIC

The difference between a mediocre workout and a brilliant one can sometimes all come down to the music you play. I have an ever-expanding playlist on my phone that I put on every time I plan to do a strenuous workout, and it never fails to make me feel happy and motivated. Choose your favourite tracks with a beat that you can keep up with, put on your runners and go!

3

GET A WORKOUT BUDDY

Let's face it – it's easy to make excuses for skipping exercise. But having a workout buddy, such as a friend, family member or partner, means you're accountable. It's harder to skip training when you have arranged to meet someone else at the gym or park. Look for someone motivated and at a similar level of fitness as you so that neither of you feel like you're at a disadvantage. If a personal trainer is a feasible option for you, then I definitely recommend it for their encouragement, advice and expertise.

4

INVEST IN NEW WORKOUT CLOTHES

I find that having colourful, fun clothes to wear for my workouts really helps to make me feel excited and motivated. It's also less pleasant to go to the gym when you're not feeling good about what you're wearing. There's a great range of brightly coloured sportswear available in shops now that doesn't cost a fortune and a decent pair of runners will make all the difference to your training experience.

5

MAKE HEALTHIER CHOICES

As I will explain in the next chapter, nutrition is the key to getting the most out of your workouts – food choices contribute to as much as 80% of your fitness results. That's huge, so your meals need to be created to keep you feeling energised and motivated. If you're not providing your body with the correct nutrients or you're eating processed foods lacking in nutrients, then your energy will likely be low and your sleep may even suffer too. Eating a balanced diet with plenty of complete sources of protein is crucial to muscle recovery and growth. Healthy complex carbs like sweet potatoes, butternut squash and oats provide the energy for training, while smoothies and fruit are good sources of quick pre-workout fuel.

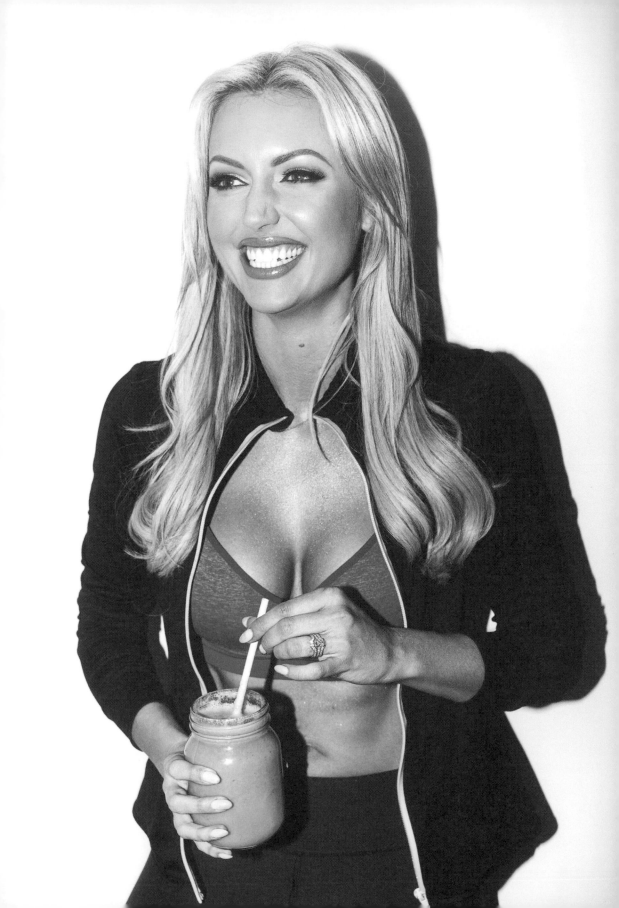

BODY CONFIDENCE TIPS

If you're a bride-to-be or aiming to get in shape to feel great for a holiday, party or big event, then you will want to feel like the best version of yourself when the big day arrives. For my own wedding in the summer of 2014, I didn't want to lose weight, but I did want to feel lean, toned, confident and healthy. I focused on following these 10 body tips in the lead-up to my big day, and they really helped me to look and feel my best.

1

AVOID REFINED SUGAR

Found in a wide range of both sweet and savoury foods, from packaged goods such as biscuits, cakes, crackers and baked treats to sweets, ice cream, sorbet, cereal, jam, yogurts, chocolate, soups, pasta sauces, breads, sweetened plant milks and fizzy drinks, refined sugar is one of the most damaging foods for your skin and body. It may even cause skin to age more quickly through a process called glycation, by which metabolised sugar molecules could damage the collagen and elastin fibres that keep skin youthful and plump.

Simple sugars provide an instant burst of energy for the body, which is why so many people reach for a biscuit or bar to combat that mid-afternoon energy slump. But this instant rush of glucose into your bloodstream causes your blood sugar to quickly rise as it triggers the pancreas to release insulin, which stores the excess glucose as fat. Insulin is a major fat-storing hormone, and its control is crucial to successful long-term weight management.

If you're somebody who battles with your weight, constantly snacks on sugary treats and suffers from energy highs and lows, then you may find yourself caught in an addictive cycle, which can be challenging to break. Refined sugar is the worst type of food you can eat if your aim is to lose body fat and boost your energy levels. It can deplete your body of vital nutrients, including magnesium, vitamin C needed for plump skin and B vitamins for energy production. It can encourage weight gain around the middle, disrupt appetite hormone regulation, triggering you to eat more, and it places unnecessary stress on your body.

It can damage the special cells of the immune system, leaving you more vulnerable to colds and other illnesses. Refined sugar may also cause your body to look and feel more bloated than normal, as glycogen is stored with molecules of water to eventually be used as energy.

The very best way to stabilise blood sugar levels to feel calm, balanced and satisfied throughout the day is by eating a diet high in fibre, lean protein, healthy fats and complex carbs.

All my recipes are free from refined sugar, are fibre rich and are designed to stabilise blood sugar levels. If you regularly eat sugary foods or add sugar to hot drinks, then my advice is to try to wean yourself off it in plenty of time before your wedding day, holiday, party or important event, as it takes around 21 days to break the habit and really feel the benefits. Get used to reading labels carefully in order to avoid added refined sugar and other processed ingredients.

2

MANAGE STRESS LEVELS

Many people are so chronically stressed out that they have begun to see it as normal. But long-term stress can be detrimental to your overall health, weight, fitness levels, emotional health and sleep patterns.

Have you heard about the connection between high stress levels and weight gain around the middle? Adrenaline is released when stress levels are raised. It increases levels of cortisol circulating in the body, which is the stress hormone that encourages fat to be stored around your middle. When you factor in the refined sugar that many people eat daily, there's a serious insulin spike to add to the cortisol levels. Together, these hormones are a disaster for anybody trying to shift stomach fat and combat bloating. As I explained, insulin is the fat-storing hormone that instructs the body to store fat around your middle to be easily accessed for quick energy. So cortisol and insulin can work together to add weight around the midsection and increase your cravings for more sugar and caffeine. It's truly a vicious cycle.

I find that taking time out each day to exercise and simply relax can really help to lower stress levels. But everybody is different and what matters most is finding the time to regularly relax and unwind. Spending time with friends and family, meditation, yoga, watching a movie, having a bath, going for a massage, cuddling your pet and reducing your caffeine intake can all help to lower those cortisol levels to help you look and feel your best.

3

BANISH BLOATING FOODS

Feeling bloated? There may be a large number of reasons why. Constipation can be an issue for many people, and is undoubtedly one of the main causes of bloating. However, eating a diet high in fibre-rich plant foods and drinking more water can make a big difference for a lot of people.

For many women, it's simply hormonal and an annoying symptom of that time of the month. For others, it can be a result of eating too quickly and gulping in excess air, not chewing food correctly, eating foods that your body may find difficult to digest and is sensitive to, or the carbon dioxide in fizzy drinks.

However, there's another reason to consider: bacterial overgrowth in the small intestine, also known as SIBO. Humans naturally have more bacteria in their bodies than actual body cells. Gut bacteria is a complex area because there are at least 500 different species of micro-flora living in the normal human gut. The

'friendly' bacteria work hard to maintain an optimal environment for food digestion and immune system health and they synthesise certain vitamins, amongst many other necessary tasks. Their job is to also keep the unfriendly bacteria, yeasts and parasites at bay. The upper section of your intestine has been designed to remain quite low in bacteria of all types, but if bacteria multiply in high amounts in the first two sections of the intestine, they may compete with you for nutrition.

SIBO remains a poorly understood issue, although bloating, excessive gas production, nausea, diarrhoea and feelings of being too full after eating may occur when bacteria or yeast reach the food in the upper intestine and ferment the carbohydrates present. Foods high in refined sugar and white flour are more prone to cause bacterial overgrowth and bloating. Some people also get very bloated from excess fructose in their diet, which impoves by avoiding sweet fruits like bananas, grapes and pineapple, as well as fruit juices, honey and many other sweet foods. A compromised immune system or a diet low in dietary fibre may also be a cause for excess bacterial growth. Always speak to your GP if you suffer from digestive issues.

All of the recipes in this book are designed to maximise your intake of fibre and build your immune system to help resist infections. One of the best ways of controlling excess bacteria and its effects is to take probiotics daily or enjoy fermented foods and drinks regularly. We're all different, so certain foods that can cause bloating for some may have no effect on others.

If you do suffer from bloating, then I encourage you to keep a food diary to try to find a link between the foods you're eating regularly and when you feel excessively bloated. I have discovered that gluten and wheat-based foods, yeast, dairy, refined sugar and salt all cause me to look and feel bloated, so I have to be careful to avoid them.

4

TAKE PROBIOTICS

I've just explained why probiotics can help control bloating, and I believe that they're one of the most important factors to introduce to your daily life in order to boost digestion and reduce digestive discomfort.

There are many benefits of probiotics. They can improve digestion, liver function, allergy resistance and B vitamin synthesis, increase overall energy, enhance nutrient absorption and help to banish bloating. Probiotics can help to improve nutrient absorption and satisfaction after meals, meaning that you're less likely to continue snacking.

5

DRINK ALCOHOL IN MODERATION

Alcohol is not a friend to your waistline. It can trigger stomach fat to build up around your mid-section because it's quickly absorbed into your bloodstream and deposited in the stomach area. That's why some heavy drinkers can develop 'beer bellies'. It may cause you to gain many unwanted pounds due in part to the hundreds of extra calories in sugary cocktails and mixers, while wine and beer are also high in sugar and calories. But alcohol itself is a simple sugar, which hits your bloodstream fast and causes insulin levels to increase, encouraging fat storage. All alcohol contains seven calories per gram, which is just under the nine calories per gram of fat. Being a liquid devoid of fibre, it doesn't make you feel full, so it can be easy to overdo it.

Drinking alcohol may also slow down your metabolism because the liver prioritises the metabolism of alcohol before it can process energy from the food you have eaten. So for a certain period of time, it may actually prevent your body from burning fat efficiently. It must stop burning off the calories from your last meal while the alcohol consumption is broken down, which can store whatever you've eaten as fat. The Irish government recommendations for alcohol consumption are up to 11 standard drinks a week for women and up to 17 standard drinks for a man.

6

DAILY GREENS

I speak at length about the importance of consuming abundant leafy greens, as calorie for calorie, they're the most nutritionally dense type of food that you can eat, packed with fibre, minerals and protective phytonutrients.

Many people find it easier to ingest them in smoothie or juice form than in a salad, which is why you'll find a number of green smoothie recipes in this book, including my signature green goddess smoothie (page 133) and green goddess juice (page 134).

Enjoying blended greens really helps to boost your complexion, hair growth and encourage a flat stomach. Your digestive system has less work to do, meaning you save precious digestive energy and the nutrients are delivered much more quickly to your cells via your bloodstream. I love to drink a protein smoothie after a workout because all the goodness goes straight to repairing torn muscle fibres and boosting your energy.

In addition, the dietary fibre remains as part of a smoothie, which is so important for a healthy digestive system and to encourage fat burning.

7

FILL UP ON LOW-CALORIE, NUTRIENT-DENSE FOODS

It makes sense that the more you fill your body with nutrient-dense foods, the more satisfied you will feel and you will hopefully be far less likely to overeat or snack on sugary foods. Sometimes those who make less healthy food choices or base their diet on processed foods can be driven to continue eating long after they're full because their body is not efficiently absorbing the variety of nutrients it needs for normal everyday function. It continues to demand food, and these hunger signals may be interpreted by the individual as a craving for fatty or sugary foods.

If you aim to base your diet on whole, nutrient-rich foods, then your body should feel far more satisfied and you will be less likely to crave junk food and sugar. Filling up on plenty of fresh fruit and veggies, healthy fats and lean protein will naturally encourage your weight to stabilise at what is ideal for your height and build.

8

EAT HEALTHY FATS

There is no need to fear fat. The right type of essential fat is important for building a smooth and soft complexion, growing glossy hair and encouraging normal hormone function, efficient fat burning, healthy brain function, eyesight and joints, and so much more. In fact, you need to eat healthy fat to help burn excess body fat.

Aim to eat fat every day from sources including avocados, nuts and seeds and their butters, coconut oil and other high-quality cold-pressed oils such as hemp seed and walnut, and organic or wild salmon if you're a fish eater.

Fat is a concentrated macronutrient, so you don't need to eat too much of it to reap its many health benefits. There are nine calories per gram of fat, which is more than double the calorie content of both protein and carbs, which both contain four calories per gram. Two tablespoons of hemp, chia or ground flaxseeds on your porridge each morning, a handful of raw walnuts as a snack or half an avocado each day are sufficient quantities. Fat can also help you to lose weight because it keeps you feeling full and satiated for a number of hours, which means you'll be less likely to snack on unhealthy foods. If I'm in a rush, I'll have a couple teaspoons of almond butter to keep me going until I can get a proper meal.

9

WEIGHT TRAIN

I've spoken about how effective weight training is for both men and women, especially if you're trying to tone up and shift some body fat before your wedding day or a holiday. Plenty of people step up their exercise regime ahead of their big day, and there are few more powerful motivations to get fit than an upcoming wedding.

I increased my workouts and upped their intensity even more in the lead-up to my wedding to help me feel my most strong and confident. It's obviously important to train all your major muscle groups each week, but as my dress had a full skirt and a fitted waist with my shoulders and arms on show, I placed plenty of focus on training my upper body. I made sure to train my chest, shoulder, triceps, biceps and back each week and did plenty of Pilates to strengthen and lengthen muscles and improve posture.

10

STAY HYDRATED

It can be surprisingly easy to go through your day without drinking enough water, not realising that you're becoming increasingly dehydrated. If you're a regular tea or coffee drinker, then too much caffeine can also contribute to dehydration.

Did you know that your body can sometimes mistake feelings of thirst for hunger? This may cause you to reach for unhealthy snacks such as biscuits or crisps. If you feel hungry between meals, drink a glass of water and wait a couple of minutes to see if it helps.

If you feel a little bloated, try drinking more water. It really helps to boost kidney function, improve lymphatic drainage and help your body to flush out toxins. Eight glasses of water a day is the normal recommendation, and more in warm weather or if you exercise regularly. Try to reduce caffeine intake too and replace caffeinated drinks with caffeine-free herbal teas. Pop a couple slices of lemon and lime or a sprig of mint into chilled water if you find the taste too plain.

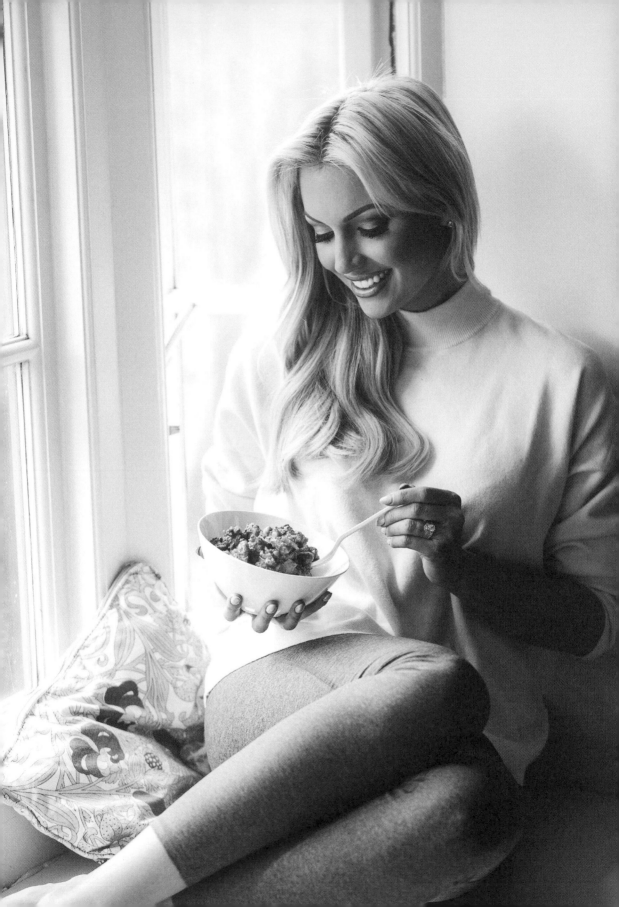

PART 3

FITNESS FOOD

"Every living cell in your body is made
from the food you eat. If you consistently eat
junk food then you'll have a junk body."

JEANETTE JENKINS

Many plants are a great source of protein, and eating a plant-based diet doesn't mean you will miss out on your body's protein requirements.

Protein is essential for fitness, fat loss and building and maintaining strong, lean muscles as well as for growth and repair in your body and for the production of transport molecules, enzymes, hormones and antibodies. It also helps to improve calcium absorption, making it an integral part of bone health. Plants come with all the amino acids you require in a nutritionally perfect package that also contains iron, calcium, antioxidants, phytochemicals and fibre, which is essential for weight loss.

An individual's protein needs will differ from day to day depending on what they're doing, so the only exact way to know the protein needs of an individual is to conduct a study of their nitrogen balance on that particular day.

The World Health Organization's protein recommendation is 5–10% of daily calories or about 0.8g protein per kg of body weight, going up to 1.2g/kg or more for active males. This translates as approximately 90g of protein a day for an active 75kg man and 48–64g for a lightly to moderately active 64kg woman, for example. On a 1,800 calorie diet, 10% protein would be 45g.

Plant foods easily contain enough protein once caloric needs are met. The average protein level in pulses is 27% of calories, in nuts and seeds it's 13% and in grains it's 12%.

AMINO ACIDS
There are nine essential amino acids that must be eaten regularly because they can't be made in your body: histidine, isoleucine, leucine, lysine, methionine, phenylalanine, threonine, tryptophan and valine.

A food that contains all nine is known as a complete protein. Like beads on a string, they form together in various sequences to build the proteins needed for the many everyday biochemical processes in your body. Your food must first be broken down into amino acids, which are then rebuilt into the protein chains specific to human muscles.

Research suggests that amino acids from plant foods are readily available to your body. A wide range of plants contain plentiful quantities of all the essential

amino acids, so it is virtually impossible for you to become protein deficient if your diet contains enough calories from whole foods.

Most plants are low in fat and rich in essential minerals, including iron and calcium. Iron is an important mineral for supporting energy levels and helping to prevent anaemia, and calcium is essential for bone health and normal muscle function. In 500 calories of tomatoes, spinach, butter beans, peas and potatoes, you will find up to 20g of iron and 545mg of calcium.

Plant foods are also packed with the antioxidant nutrient beta-carotene, which is known to boost and brighten the complexion, slow down the ageing process and mop up damaging free radicals in your system. Carrots, sweet potatoes and butternut squash owe their vibrant orange colour to beta-carotene, which in turn brings colour and radiance to your skin.

BUILDING MUSCLE WITH PLANT FOOD
There are so many valuable sources of complete plant-based protein built into a nutrient-rich package to help shed extra pounds, boost your health and maximise the benefits of your workouts.

Lentils and beans are a staple in my diet and appear in plenty of my recipes, as they're an excellent source of inexpensive and complete plant protein, antioxidants, fibre, vitamins and minerals. I love to sprout lentils, chickpeas, broccoli seeds, alfalfa and adzuki beans in my own kitchen, but I'm also a fan of cooked beans and legumes. They're ideal for adding satisfying warmth and density to your diet without having to worry about weight gain, as beans are naturally low in fat and high in fibre. In addition, they're high in minerals like iron, calcium and magnesium, plus vitamins and phytonutrients to help prevent the signs of ageing.

Protein powders have become hugely popular with gym-goers in the past few years, yet many commercial protein powders contain preservatives, genetically modified ingredients, whey and soy protein isolates, which can be a problem for those sensitive to soy. Some may also contain chemical sweeteners like aspartame and saccharin. A good-quality hemp or pea protein powder or the Sunwarrior brand of raw plant-based protein powders are my top recommendations for adding to a smoothie or shake to boost post-weights muscle recovery. Sunwarrior is a good option because it's raw, unprocessed, sweetened with stevia and is free from gluten, soy and dairy, with 15g of protein and just 80 calories per serving.

Green vegetables come in a nutritionally perfect package of fibre, phytonu-trients, minerals, vitamins, antioxidants and essential fatty acids. By focusing on vegetables in each meal, you will be benefiting from the fibre, antioxidant vitamins and phytonutrients that meat, poultry and eggs lack while also lessening the amount of cholesterol you consume.

Eaten raw, nuts, seeds and their butters are a super source of plant protein. However, they are a dense food, so about a handful a day is generally enough, or a little more if you're extremely active or trying to gain weight. Shops and supermarkets are full of roasted and salted nuts and seeds, but nuts will benefit your health most when eaten in their natural, unsalted state. Roasting them can denature their amino acids and destroy their healthy fatty acids, plus they're often cooked in unhealthy vegetable oils.

Fitness foods

Following a diet rich in whole foods and avoiding excessive alcohol and smoking helps you to benefit most from your fitness regime. Choosing the right type of foods to eat before and after a workout, and in general to support an active lifestyle, is key to ensuring you look and feel your very best and that you get the most out of your exercise regime.

Whole, unprocessed foods contain an array of vitamins, minerals, antioxidants and amino acids, ready to be absorbed and assimilated into your body to repair and rebuild torn muscle fibres after a tough workout. I've designed the recipes in this book to be rich in essential amino acids from different sources to ensure that you're getting the complete range for your body's daily needs. Protein also helps to keep you feeling full, which means you'll be less likely to snack on sugary or fatty foods.

These are my favourite fitness foods for building muscle tone, reducing body fat and boosting energy levels.

QUINOA

Originating from South America, quinoa is actually a seed rather than a grain and is naturally gluten free. With over 8g of protein per cup (cooked), it contains all the essential amino acids plus fibre and minerals including manganese, phosphorus, copper and magnesium. It's also a good source of antioxidant phytonutrients, including quercetin. These protect your cells from free radical damage and accelerated ageing.

LENTILS

These tiny nutrient powerhouses are high in fibre, low in fat and packed with antioxidants and essential minerals. They contain an impressive 18g of protein per cup (cooked). Lentils are so simple to cook with and I love to use them in soups, salads, curries and stews.

HEMP SEEDS

One of the very best sources of complete plant-based protein, which also have the perfect balance of omega-6 to omega-3 fats to help keep your skin smooth and plump, hemp seeds are incredibly versatile. They're also one of the best foods for building lean muscle and work well sprinkled onto smoothies, salads, steamed veggies and soups.

BEANS

Beans are a staple in my diet as they're so versatile and come in a wide range of varieties. With 12–15g of protein per cup, they're a brilliant muscle-building, fat-loss food as they're low in fat and calories but high in fibre, vitamins and minerals such as iron, calcium and zinc. My favourites include chickpeas, kidney beans, butter beans and black beans.

SPIRULINA

It may taste very 'green', but this microalgae is an incredible source of easily absorbed protein. In fact, spirulina boasts a whopping 60% protein, which makes it the highest of any naturally found food. It's a powerful food and it's easy to incorporate into your daily diet. I often add a small spoonful into my green goddess smoothie (page 133) and it boosts the nutrient value of my supergreen smoothie bowl (page 106).

NUTRITIONAL YEAST

Nutritional yeast is an inactive form of yeast and an absolute staple for plant-based diets. It's similar to Parmesan cheese in that it instantly adds a nutty, cheesy flavour to foods like soups and sauces, plus I sprinkle it over salads. It's also highly nutritious – a 2 tablespoon serving offers 7g of protein in the form of all the essential amino acids, plus iron, fibre and a range of B vitamins. Some brands are fortified with zinc and vitamin B12.

Pre-workout foods for energy

It's important to eat for energy around 45–60 minutes before a workout. I often opt for a green goddess smoothie (page 133) and a handful of raw almonds for a great combination of easily digested protein, fat, fibre and carbs.

Smoothies work so well for boosting energy because the nutrients have been released from the plant cell and are available to be quickly absorbed into your blood for instant, clean-burning energy that won't send insulin levels skyward. They free up digestive energy, which will benefit your workout, as it's best to avoid anything that's difficult to digest or makes you feel sluggish. If you're in a rush, then a simple sliced banana or apple with a couple teaspoons of nut butter makes a speedy and energy-boosting snack.

Post-workout foods for muscle repair

Post-workout nourishment is crucial for recovery, as this is the time to replace used-up glycogen stores to replenish your liver and muscles. Try to eat within 30–45 minutes of finishing up exercise, as this is the time period during which your body most urgently requires nutrients.

After weight training, you need protein to begin the process of healing and rebuilding torn muscle, as this is how you tone and strengthen muscles to get more toned over time. But intense exercise also releases free radicals into circulation, which can contribute to cellular damage and premature ageing. It's really important to eat antioxidant-rich foods after a workout to help protect your cells.

Protein smoothies are an excellent option post-workout, as they don't require much digestion and their nutrients are delivered quickly to muscles and tissues to begin the process of rebuilding and repairing. I often make my blue warrior recovery shake (page 136) after a tough weights workout, as it contains an ideal combination of digestible raw plant protein, anti-inflammatory omega-3 fats, high-fibre carbs and a rich assortment of antioxidants from the blueberries.

I usually bring a smoothie with me to drink straight after training, then enjoy a balanced meal once I'm home, containing protein, complex carbs and healthy fats.

Foods to build abs

Strong, visible abdominal muscles are one of the most popular areas of the body for developing. Not only do they help to create a visually healthy and fit physique, but having a strong core helps to improve your posture, protect your body from injury and really helps with every other type of physical movement.

Hours of crunches aren't going to give you a visible six-pack, though. We all have abdominal muscles, but the number one key to making them visible is a 'clean' diet. Sufficient cardiovascular exercise helps to burn body fat, while abs and core exercises help to strengthen and build the muscles. Ever heard the expression 'abs are made in the kitchen, not the gym'?

The best foods for building abs are natural, whole foods, low in simple carbs and high in amino acids, fibre, essential fats, vitamins and minerals.

These are the foods I focus on for meals and snacks when I want to strip back body fat and build up my abs:

Almonds and almond butter
Avocados
Berries
Broccoli
Chickpeas
Hemp seeds
Leafy green vegetables
Lentils
Nutritional yeast
Quinoa
Sweet potatoes
Vegan protein powder

How to lose body fat

Want to look lean, toned and fit? The key to looking and feeling fit is to keep body fat levels down while maintaining and building lean muscle mass. This means that your muscles, especially your abs, will become more visible.

The right balance needs to be struck between eating enough calories and the correct nutrients to fuel your body and repair muscles without allowing your body to store excess as fat. You must optimise your metabolism while keeping blood sugar levels and insulin stable and you must never allow your body to go hungry, as it may slow down your metabolic rate if it senses a period of starvation.

The most powerful and effective way to slim down and stay lean, healthy and fit for life is to base your diet on high-fibre whole plant foods, complete protein sources and a smaller amount of calorie-dense foods, such as healthy fats.

Greatly reducing or totally eliminating refined sugar, white flour, processed foods, vegetable oils, shop-bought salad dressings and sauces, fizzy drinks, alcohol and fried foods while keeping active and watching portion sizes will help to stabilise your body weight at what is healthy, happy and ideal for your height, age, gender and activity levels.

You can tone up different parts of your body, but you cannot spot-reduce body fat from specific areas such as your tummy or thighs, nor can you lose or gain more than two pounds of body fat per week. Any extra will be water weight or muscle.

Restrictive quick-fix diets that dramatically reduce carbs and calories may work in the very short term because you're draining your muscles of stored carbs (glycogen), which reduces water weight and excess bloating. But they don't work in the long term or as a lifestyle solution because they're neither sustainable nor healthy.

When embarking on a weight loss plan, it becomes even more crucial that everything you put into your body is rich in nutrients so that no deficiencies can arise. That's one of the many reasons I don't recommend packaged, processed diet meals and snacks and base all my recipes on whole foods. A deficiency in certain nutrients and amino acids may trigger low moods and severe cravings for sugar, which must be avoided for successful weight loss.

CALORIE COUNTING

I don't believe in calorie counting under normal circumstances because it can be tedious and time consuming and can remove the focus from the importance of healthy whole foods. I much prefer to concentrate on eating nutrient-dense foods over calorie-dense foods, practising portion control, avoiding refined sugar and only eating until I'm three-quarters full. Listening to the hunger and satiety signals from your own body is key to maintaining a healthy and normal weight.

However, calories do matter when it comes to body fat loss and it's pretty much an exact science, which makes it easier to navigate. One pound of fat is equal to 3,500 calories. So to lose one pound of fat a week, you must either eat 500 fewer calories a day or burn them through exercise. Either option alone is challenging, which is why combining exercise with calorie counting will achieve the best results. This is a steady and sustainable goal that can be safely followed over a longer period of time.

If you require faster results, then you could increase this weight loss to two pounds a week by applying the same mathematics to eat less or burn off 1,000 calories a day. Time-wise, it's generally more practical for most people to eat less rather than spend hours exercising, which makes this degree of weight loss challenging. It's also not as safe and sustainable in the long term because you would have to cut calories dramatically down from what you're used to while still getting all the nutrients you require and maintaining consistent, intense exercise.

CALCULATE YOUR BASAL METABOLIC RATE

Before you begin a weight loss programme, it's necessary to calculate your basal metabolic rate (BMR). This depends on your height, weight, age, gender and activity levels. It calculates the minimum number of calories your body needs simply to stay alive if you're completely sedentary, even sleeping. It decreases with age and lower muscle mass, and increases as you gain muscle.

After that, you will need to account for your physical activity levels, as the calories you burn will need to be calculated. For example, my BMR is 1,400 calories and I would be considered moderately active, so I burn up to 1,820 calories per day. To lose one pound of body fat a week, I need to consume 1,320 calories a day, which is a deficit of 500 per day and 3,500 per week.

I strongly recommend you use an app or website to calculate your own personal calorie needs based on your BMR, as we all have individual requirements. Two of my favourites are cronometer.com and MyFitnessPal, which are free, detailed, accurate and user friendly. Any time I have had to lose a few pounds, I've followed this programme for three to four weeks, and the *Eat Yourself Fit* plan is based on my own recommended daily intake of about 1,300 calories for a weight loss of one pound per week. This is a sustainable, realistic and achievable goal, as it's important to never eat fewer than 1,200 calories a day because you may face nutrient deficiencies that can inhibit your long-term weight loss goals.

Once you calculate your numbers, you may want to adapt my plan to include slightly more or less calories. You can do this by bulking it out with more healthy fats, such as avocado or nuts, or by reducing portion sizes. But never drastically cut calories and never allow yourself to go hungry, as that will work against your health, fitness and long-term weight management.

It depends on your goals and timeline, but I strongly advise you to give yourself plenty of time to lose weight for a wedding, holiday or big event. It's safer and more achievable, as you will be losing body fat rather than water weight and muscle. In my experience, it takes eight to 12 weeks to see tangible results in your weight and body shape following a calorie-controlled healthy eating and fitness plan.

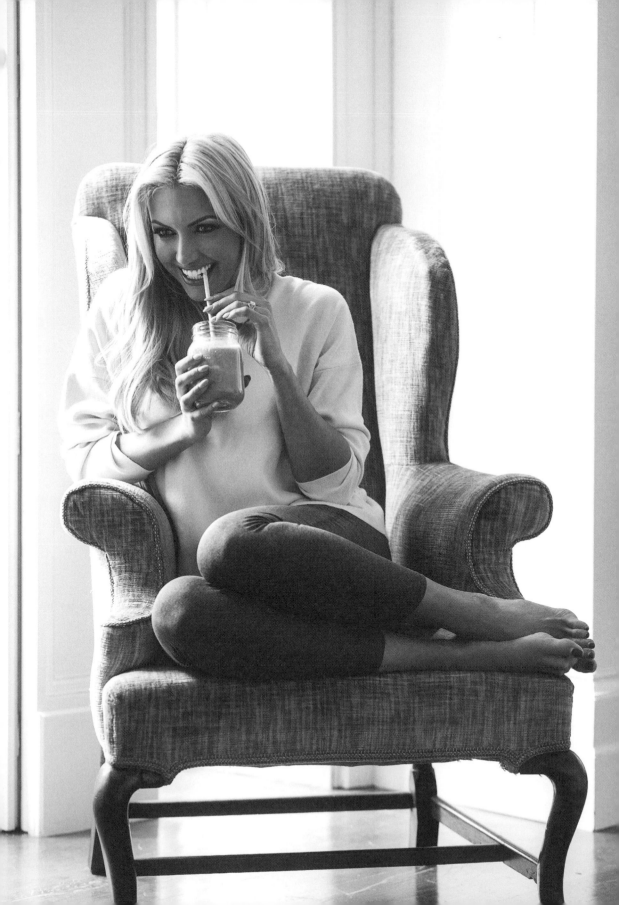

HERE ARE MY FIVE QUICK TIPS FOR LOSING BODY FAT

1

WATCH CALORIES AND PORTION SIZES

The healthy eating movement of the past few years has benefitted people in so many ways, though I think many people still struggle with weight loss, even when they're eating 'clean'. Healthy food can still contain plenty of calories, so you must be careful when replacing processed snacks with nuts and nut butters or adding avocado and dressing to salads, as their calories can quickly add up.

Do you find calorie counting tedious? Another useful way to lose weight is to use your hands for portion control. In a main meal, your serving of protein, such as beans, should be roughly the size of your palm; your serving of grains or carbs, such as sweet potato, should be the size of your fist; your portion of low-carb veggies and salad should be at least the size of your cupped hands together; and your serving of healthy fat or dressing should be about the size of your thumb.

2

LIMIT OR ELIMINATE ALCOHOL

My advice is to really limit or eliminate alcohol if you're serious about weight loss and fitness because alcohol is one of the worst substances you can consume for storing fat, especially around your middle. Add in the sugary mixers and the higher sugar content in wine and beer, and it becomes impossible to drink regularly if weight loss is your goal. It also slows down your metabolism and the yeast in certain drinks may encourage candida overgrowth. If you must have a drink, choose clear spirits with a low-sugar mixer, such as vodka with soda water and fresh lime juice.

3

AVOID SUGAR

Like alcohol, refined sugar, white flour and other simple carbs can make weight loss very difficult. They raise blood sugar levels and insulin, encouraging excess calories to be quickly stored as fat. For more effective fat loss, reduce your intake of sweet fruit, dried fruit and natural sweeteners, including maple syrup and honey. Berries are a better option to satisfy a sweet tooth.

4

GET ACTIVE

It's very difficult to achieve sustainable, healthy body fat loss without exercise. Keeping active helps to burn excess calories and build up lean muscle mass to boost your resting metabolic rate. I find that a combination of weight training and cardio really works to build muscle while burning body fat, but it's important to do what you enjoy and can fit into your lifestyle.

5

EAT SMALL MEALS REGULARLY

To encourage your metabolism to function optimally, try eating five or six smaller meals each day and aim to eat every three or four hours. This ensures that your blood sugar levels remain stable throughout the day and your body is fed a consistent stream of amino acids and other nutrients to support energy levels, muscle repair and a good mood.

HOW TO BOOST YOUR METABOLISM

Metabolism is the means by which your body converts what you eat and drink into energy. During this complex biochemical process, calories in food and beverages are combined with oxygen to release the energy your body needs to function. Even when you're sitting still or fast asleep, your body needs energy for functions such as breathing, heartbeat and blood circulation, hormone production, and growing and healing cells.

1

GET AN EARLY NIGHT

It's not always easy to get your full requirement of sleep each night, especially with work, family or study demands. But if your aim is to maintain your weight or lose a few pounds, then getting enough sleep each night is really important for a healthy and properly functioning metabolism.

It's actually pretty normal for sleep-deprived people to find that they gain an extra few pounds without changing their diet, as a lack of sleep can lead to various metabolic issues. It can cause you to burn fewer overall calories, run into problems with appetite control and experience an increase in cortisol levels, which encourages the body to store fat around the middle. Lack of sufficient sleep, which tends to be between seven and nine hours for most people, may also impair glucose tolerance, which is your body's ability to utilise sugar for fuel.

2

EAT ENOUGH PROTEIN

Firstly, your body expends more energy digesting protein than fat or carbohydrates. When you eat fat, only about 5% of the calories are used to break down that food, but when you eat protein, it's closer to 20–30%. All three major macronutrients are essential to a healthy metabolism, but eating some protein alongside complex carbs, such as oats, sweet potato, brown rice and quinoa, and healthy fats such as nuts, seeds or avocado with every meal also helps to repair and build torn muscle fibres.

Another key reason why protein is so essential to a healthy metabolic rate is because the amino acid tyrosine is a major component in the production of the thyroid hormone, thyroxine. Your thyroid controls the metabolism of every cell in your body. If you're not eating enough protein for your body's metabolic requirement, then tyrosine may be used for other functions.

Your body can recognise this as a famine state, sending out an alarm to your body to slow down its metabolic rate to store calories for survival. This is why crash dieting does not work in the long term and may even damage your metabolism. While certain vitamins and minerals can be stored in the body, amino acids must be eaten each day, and ideally in every meal and snack. But if you're eating enough calories a day from whole unprocessed foods, it's virtually impossible to become deficient in protein.

3

EAT SEA VEGETABLES

Sea vegetables, such as nori, kelp, kombu, dulse and wakame, are rich in iodine.

Iodine is an essential mineral for your thyroid health, as thyroxine is formed from iodine and the amino acid tyrosine. Without plentiful supplies of thyroxine, your thyroid can begin to dysfunction, which makes you more prone to weight gain, dry skin, fatigue, irritability and feeling constantly cold.

A notable exception to this is in the case of Hashimoto's thyroiditis, in which extra iodine may cause further health problems. If you suspect that you may have a sluggish or overactive thyroid, I advise you to book a blood test with your GP. While regular table salt generally has added iodine, I prefer to avoid refined salt and salty foods. Instead I get all the iodine I need for a healthy metabolism from sea veggies, which also add a subtle saltiness to foods. One great way to do this is to use toasted nori sheets instead of a wrap for a low-carb, high-nutrient snack or light lunch.

4

PUMP IRON

Weight or resistance training is incredibly important for strengthening all your muscles and for increasing your ratio of lean muscle to fat mass. This in turn boosts your metabolism as it encourages the body to burn calories for hours after the session while your torn muscle fibres repair themselves. Muscle at rest also burns more calories than fat.

Candida

Candida albicans is a single-celled fungus that is always found in a healthy digestive tract and genital area. Under normal circumstances it helps your body to digest and absorb nutrients, and your friendly gut bacteria help to keep it under control. But if it's allowed to multiply and grow in disproportionate amounts, it can cause infection, both locally as thrush or throughout your entire system.

There are various reasons for developing candidiasis, from a highly stressful lifestyle, overuse of antibiotics and the oral contra-ceptive pill to a diet high in processed and refined foods, especially sugars.

Candida tends to be under-diagnosed, as its symptoms may relate to a variety of other ailments. It may contribute to weight gain and gas or bloating, and it can also cause fungal infections of your skin and nails. There are some laboratory tests available for diagnosing it, including blood, stool and urine tests, so please speak to your GP if you're concerned.

Many people have had good success by overhauling their diet. Candida lives off sugar, which means that you feed it any time you eat sugar or drink alcohol, especially drinks such as wine and beer.

It can take up to six months to see symptoms disappear completely but if you follow a strict sugar-free diet, symptoms should start to noticeably improve within a number of weeks. This means following an eating plan with no refined sugar, bread, white flour-based foods, yeast-based foods, alcohol, sweet fruit, dried fruit, fruit juices or sweeteners like maple syrup and honey. I know this sounds like torture, but it should make a significant difference.

As the candida in your system begins to clear up, it's normal to experience symptoms similar to detox, including aching joints, headaches and fatigue. You may still crave sugar as the fungus is fighting to survive, but once you get through the initial first few days, the cravings subside.

Many of my *Eat Yourself Fit* recipes are devised to discourage and fight candida while encouraging the growth of healthy bacteria in your gut. However, most of my sweet treats, desserts and smoothies contain fruit, dried fruit and sweeteners, which are all free from refined sugar, but may continue to feed the candida. Generally, following a sugar-free and starch-free diet for one to three months will clear up candida. Then you can slowly start reintroducing sweet fruits and the occasional glass of wine, but reverting back to your previous high-sugar diet may cause the symptoms to return. It's also important to look after your gut health during this time by eating plenty of high-fibre veggies and taking a daily probiotic capsule after your evening meal.

I had my own struggles with candida for the very first time after my wedding and honeymoon, which led to swift weight gain and a sore, stubborn fungal infection in my nail bed.

I went on a sugar-free and alcohol-free diet and felt very tired for the first few days. I got pretty bad sugar cravings at the beginning, which I was able to handle by dabbing a pinch of ground cinnamon on the middle of my tongue (a useful trick!). Making hot chocolate with raw cacao powder, almond milk and a few drops of liquid stevia really helped me too.

I persevered and it all cleared up within six weeks. My weight naturally stabilised too. I was able to reintroduce sweeter fruits, but I avoid refined sugar and wine now as they just don't react well with me.

Sugar addiction

Experts believe that refined sugar is more addictive than cocaine because it stimulates the reward centre of your brain to release dopamine, which makes you want to experience that feeling more and more, encouraging a vicious cycle.

Refined sugar is found in almost all packaged and processed foods, even many savoury ones. Three hundred years ago, the average person ate a maximum of about 4lb of sugar per year. Now it's estimated that many people are eating close to 40 times that. A 2014 study by the National Center for Biotechnology Information in the US demonstrated that up to 75% of commercial foods and drinks contain added refined sugar.

You don't need sugar in your life and the cycle of sugar addiction can be broken. To preserve your health, waistline and skin and to keep it looking young for as long as possible, I strongly advise you to either totally eliminate refined sugar or dramatically reduce it from your diet.

MY TIPS FOR ELIMINATING SUGAR

1

GIVE IT 21 DAYS

Twenty-one days is generally considered the appropriate length of time to break a habit. I find that total abstinence for this time is the best way to break the addiction, because even tasting a little bit of sugar can kick start the cycle all over again. After just a few weeks off it, refined sugar will taste synthetic and far too sweet.

2

READ NUTRITION LABELS

Always check the ingredients listed on packaged foods carefully and never believe the hype and marketing claims made on packaging. Aim to stock up on foods as close to their natural state as possible, such as fruit, vegetables, nuts, nut butters, seeds, quinoa, beans and legumes.

3

KEEP A FOOD DIARY

This can really help you to track and eliminate mindless snacking and where and when you're adding extra sugar to your diet, such as in cups of tea and coffee or late-night cravings for sweet foods.

4

STAY HYDRATED

It can be easy to go through a busy day and forget to drink water. Get into the habit of sipping from a large bottle of water throughout the day. You need at least eight glasses of water per day and more in warm weather or if you're exercising. Veggie juices and herbal teas count too, but caffeinated drinks act as diuretics and can dehydrate you.

5

BE PREPARED

Stock up on healthy snacks. When a sugar craving hits, try eating a piece of ripe fruit with a little nut butter or a handful of raw almonds. Green apples, citrus fruits and berries are lower in sugar than other types of fruit and make a great snack.

6

CHOOSE HOMEMADE OVER EATING OUT

This can be tricky for anyone out all day at work, but being in control of what goes onto your plate can make all the difference. Aim to pack your own lunches rather than grabbing a shop-bought sandwich. Get into the habit of requesting potentially sugar-laden sauces, dips and dressings on the side and try not to tempt yourself with the bread basket or dessert menu.

7

STOCK UP ON CINNAMON

I sprinkle this sweet warming spice on a range of dishes and add it to smoothies because I find it brilliant for helping to curb sugar cravings. Plus it helps to fight fungal infections, boosts blood circulation and it's a rich source of minerals and antioxidants. It's also a good source of the mineral chromium, which helps to regulate blood sugar levels and the laying down of fat in your body.

8

CHEAT WITH A TREAT

No matter what type of eating plan you follow, if any, I think it's important to reward healthy living with an occasional tasty dessert or sweet treat. All my desserts and sweet treat recipes are simple to make and free from refined sugar, trans-fats, artificial ingredients, gluten and dairy.

ARTIFICIAL SWEETENERS

Artificial sweeteners include aspartame, saccharin and sucralose. While all have been approved and declared safe for consumption by humans, controversy remains about the potential health risks associated with these sweeteners.

Although aspartame contains no calories, detailed studies have revealed that those drinking one to two cans of fizzy diet drinks per day had a 54.5% risk of becoming overweight. This is because the phenylalanine and aspartic acid contained in aspartame may cause the release of insulin, which disrupts the hormones that control fat storage in the body. While it's one of the essential amino acids, phenylalanine acts as a neurotoxin and overexcites brain neurons when consumed in high amounts. There are high amounts of isolated phenylalanine found in aspartame, and this can lower levels of serotonin, which we know is an important neurotransmitter that helps prevent cravings for sweet and starchy foods.

Saccharin consumption may lead to more weight gain and increased levels of body fat than eating exactly the same foods sweetened with regular sugar.

AGAVE SYRUP

Agave syrup has been promoted heavily as a natural and healthy alternative to chemical sweeteners. However, it is still processed. The means by which agave is processed is almost the same as how high-fructose corn syrup is produced from cornstarch, which may cause damage to health.

The small amounts of fructose found in fruit don't cause a problem in the body, plus their high fibre and water content reduces the concentration. But in the considerable levels found in agave, it may place a strain on the liver. This is because the GI tract doesn't absorb fructose that well, so it's transported straight to the liver. Fatty liver disease, obesity and a number of other health issues have been associated with the consumption of high levels of fructose. Honey contains fructose too, so it is best eaten in moderation.

RECOMMENDED SWEETENERS

Stevia is a natural herbal sweetener that comes in a liquid or powdered form and is calorie free. It won't raise blood sugar levels or cause weight gain. It can be used to sweeten hot drinks and smoothies and you can use it in baking and in desserts too.

Xylitol is another acceptable option, and again it does not affect blood sugar levels. Cinnamon is a good sweetener because it's naturally sweet and warming, and high-quality, organic maple syrup is another sweetener I use in quite a number of my dessert recipes, as it has such a rich flavour. Although it's not raw as it has to be heat treated, it's still less processed than agave and it contains some B vitamins, calcium, magnesium, zinc and potassium.

Another good choice is organic dried fruit, once it's free from added sugar, sulphites and other preservatives. However, dried fruit is better eaten in moderation as it is higher in sugar. Dates, raisins and figs also contain a number of beneficial vitamins and minerals, including potassium, calcium, magnesium, B vitamins, copper and iron. There have been many times that dried fruit has saved me from a craving for something naughty and sweet, so it's a good idea to keep some stocked in your cupboards!

Crash diets don't work

I'm frequently asked for the quickest way to shed pounds in a week or two before a holiday, wedding or big event. A few days of eating really clean, healthy whole fruits and veggies and drinking plenty of water can definitely help to prep your stomach for a holiday as you're just helping your body to shift any stored water retention. But in the long term, those restrictive diets simply don't work.

Research shows that when you diet, blood levels of tryptophan and subsequent levels of brain serotonin drop significantly. Your brain then demands that you eat carbohydrates immediately, and the message is so powerful that even the strongest-willed person would probably struggle to ignore it. If your diet is also low in nutrients, including zinc and vitamin B6, then a similar craving for stodgy carbs may arise because you'll likely be failing to produce sufficient serotonin.

Depending on the person, these low-serotonin cravings can range from fancying a biscuit with a cup of tea to a full-blown binge on bread, chocolate, ice cream, crisps, chips and whatever else you can get your hands on. This is why the majority of diets do not work!

YO-YO DIETING AND THE SET POINT THEORY

Yo-yo dieting may be tempting as a quick fix, but it generally does more harm than good. Dieters find themselves on a constant roller coaster of weight loss and weight gain, often gaining back even more than they originally weighed. It can become a constant, stressful and soul-destroying cycle.

The set point theory may explain why dieters end up exceeding their original weight with rebound overeating. The 'set point' is the weight that your body tries to keep at a steady level by regulating the amount of food and calories eaten. Research shows that each person has a programmed 'set point' weight, controlled by your individual fat cells. When the fat cell begins to shrink as the person diets, it sends a strong message to the brain, telling it to eat immediately as the body is facing a starvation state.

The set point is yet another explanation as to why calorie-restricting diets don't work, and certainly not in the long term. A person determined to lose weight is able to use sheer willpower in the short term to fight off the urge to eat what they normally do, but the impulse usually becomes too powerful to ignore. What follows is 'rebound eating', and the person frequently ends up gaining more weight than before. This reprogrammes their set point to an even higher level, making future weight loss even tougher.

SO WHAT'S THE ANSWER?

The big secret to overriding the set point in your fat cells is to increase your insulin sensitivity to enable fat stores to be burned for energy. How do you do this? By exercising regularly, eating a high-fibre, whole-foods diet full of veggies, fruit, beans and legumes, nuts and seeds, and trying to avoid blood sugar-raising foods and drinks, including refined sugar, soft drinks, alcohol, white flour, fruit juice, chips, crisps and other junk foods.

MY TOP 10 FOODS FOR FAT LOSS

These are my top 10 favourite foods to focus on for helping fat loss and boosting overall health, and they crop up in most of my recipes.

1

KALE

Kale is part of the brassica family. It has a mellow, earthy taste and its large, waxy leaves provide more nutritional value for fewer calories than almost any other food available. It's rich in fibre and water to keep you feeling full, to boost fat burning, to maintain a healthy digestive system and to make you less likely to overeat, plus it has an abundance of essential vitamins, minerals and disease-fighting antioxidant compounds. Kale contains a concentration of two types of important antioxidants, called carotenoids and flavonoids. Calorie for calorie, it contains more calcium than milk, more iron than beef, 10% more vitamin C than spinach and is high in amino acids, antioxidants, vitamins A and E and minerals.

2

CHICKPEAS

Chickpeas are an excellent fat loss and fitness food to include in your diet regularly. They're low fat, rich in complete protein and B vitamins to boost energy levels and support a healthy metabolism, and they're packed with fibre to encourage normal digestive health and banish bloating. They're also lower in starch than many other types of beans, so they're easier to digest and they help to keep blood sugar levels stable.

3

LENTILS

Fibre is essential for weight loss and effective fat burning, as it fills you up, boosts your metabolism and contains no calories. Lentils are full of fibre, with almost 12g per cup (cooked). They're also low in calories, high in protein and iron and they contain virtually zero fat. The perfect fitness food.

4

BERRIES

Nature's sweet treats in a perfect package! Berries are amongst the fruit lowest in sugar and calories, and they contain plenty of fibre to keep blood sugar levels and insulin stable. Rich in antioxidants, they assist in reducing inflammation in the body, protect your skin from the early signs of ageing and help to banish sugar cravings.

5

SWEET POTATOES

A great source of complex carbs, sweet potatoes are low calorie, with virtually no fat and plenty of fibre to keep you feeling satisfied between meals. They don't raise blood sugar in the same way that regular potatoes do, making them a reliable and versatile fat-loss food.

6

PLANT-BASED PROTEIN POWDER

Protein is so important for burning body fat, as it requires more energy for your body to digest and helps build lean muscle to keep you toned and slim. Hemp powder and other forms of raw, vegan protein powder are excellent sources of complete protein without having excess calories. They also work well in smoothies and protein bars and balls.

7

CHIA SEEDS

These tiny seeds can absorb liquid and swell up to 15 times their size, making them a brilliant food for weight loss as they keep you feeling full for hours. With high levels of protein and fibre, chia seeds are also one of the very best sources of omega-3 fats to nourish your skin and help keep your cell membranes strong and supple.

8

ALMONDS AND ALMOND BUTTER

Not only are they a good source of easily assimilated plant protein, but raw unsalted almonds are one of the very best food sources of vitamin E to nourish, soften and protect your skin from sun damage. Opt for a handful a day to snack on between meals as they help to stabilise blood sugar levels. Raw almond butter is a great way to enjoy these protein-rich nuts, but aim for no more than a tablespoon per day.

9

QUINOA

This naturally gluten-free seed is packed with fibre, complete protein, magnesium, B vitamins, iron and potassium to boost energy and support weight loss and fitness goals. It's higher in amino acids and minerals and lower in carbs than couscous or rice.

10

OATMEAL

Oats are simple to prepare and fill you up quickly, helping to keep blood sugar and insulin levels stable. They're also higher in protein than many other grains, lower in non-fibre carbs and rich in energy-boosting B vitamins. The beta-glucans in oatmeal help to lower bad cholesterol by removing it from the bloodstream.

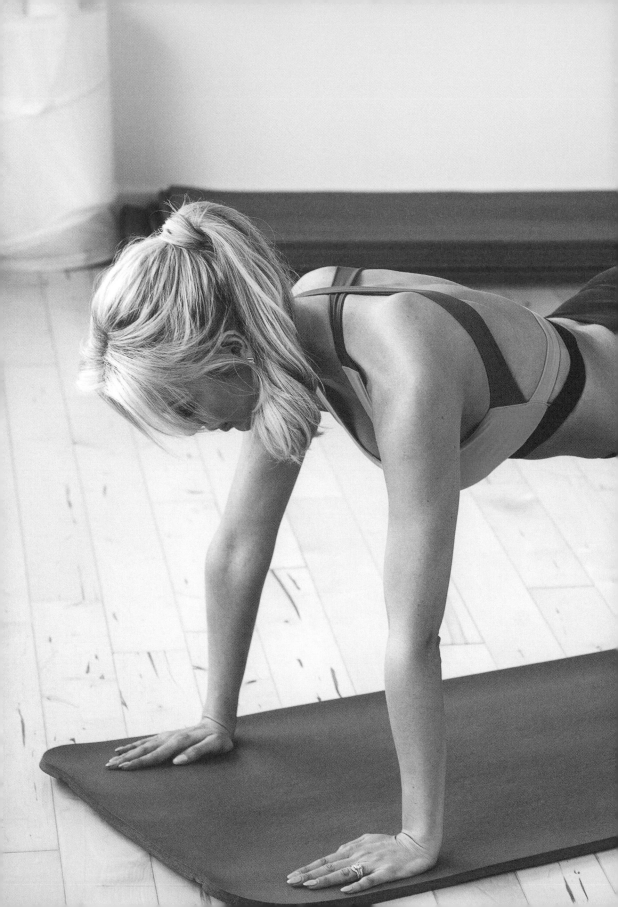

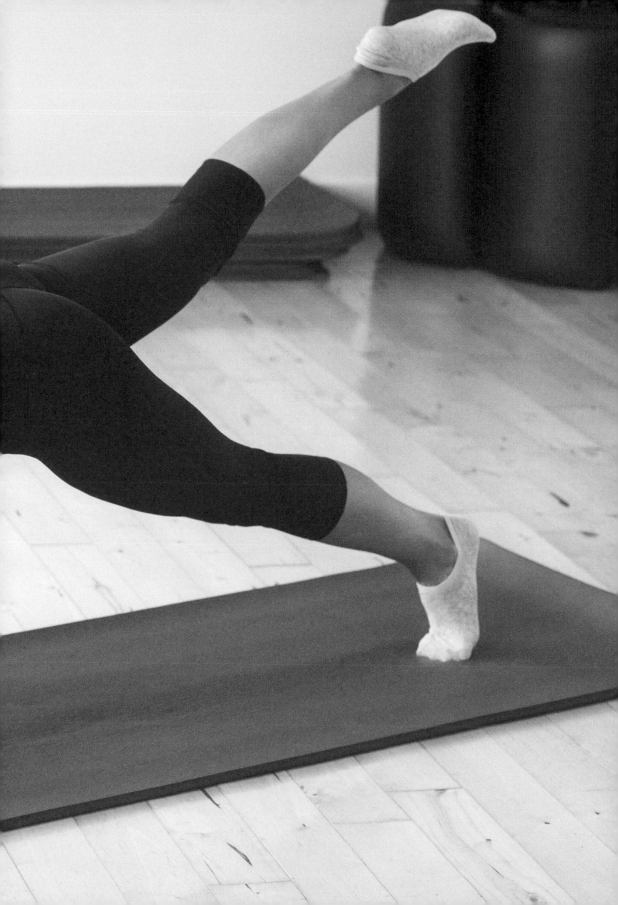

Appetite control

Do you ever have days or weeks when you feel hungry all the time and no amount of food can satiate you? There can be a number of reasons involved in that feeling of being full enough to stop eating, so it's important to get used to listening to your body's hunger and satiety signals.

Food portions served in restaurants tend to be much bigger than they ought to be, and people often think that they need more food than they really do. This can lead to overeating and taking in more calories than the body can burn, which encourages fat storage over time.

If you find yourself constantly snacking and would like to take steps to break the cycle, ask yourself these four questions.

ARE YOU GENUINELY HUNGRY?
One of the most effective ways to gain control of your weight for life is to really pay attention to what your body is telling you. It's easy to get into the habit of eating out of boredom or emotional eating if you're feeling upset or lonely. I've always encouraged clients I've worked with for weight loss to ask themselves if they're really hungry before they reach for a snack.

ARE YOU PROPERLY HYDRATED?
Try drinking a glass of water first and waiting a few minutes to see if you're still peckish. Caffeinated drinks like tea, coffee and some fizzy drinks will act as a diuretic and cause more water to be expelled from your body, which can lead to dehydration. Herbal teas can help if you're looking for a slightly sweeter taste. Try adding a few drops of liquid stevia to sweeten them even more.

ARE YOU EATING ON THE RUN?
Slowing down, being present in the moment and really developing your awareness around food, snacking and the relationship between food and your body can make all the difference when it comes to achieving your ideal weight.

We lead busy, demanding lives, so eating on the run is something we can all be guilty of. But making less healthy choices when out and about and then gulping down food can really impact on your waistline and digestion. I keep a packet of raw almonds in my handbag so that I always have a healthy snack on hand to keep me going until I can eat a proper meal.

ARE YOU FEELING FULL?
Putting down your knife and fork when you're three-quarters full is my favourite tip for portion control on a plant-based diet, and it means that counting calories isn't necessary. Low-fat plant-based meals are nutrient dense but low in calorific energy, so you would have to feel seriously stuffed before you overdo it on excess energy. Listening to your body and appetite signals, eating from a smaller plate and finishing when you're three-quarters full

will ensure that your weight will stabilise to what is ideal for your body type and height.

For many people, eating five or six small meals a day and never going for longer than three to four hours without food can help to balance their blood sugar levels, preventing extreme hunger and the urge to binge on calorie-rich foods.

The stomach stretch response

One key reason for being tempted to overeat is linked to the actual stretch and feeling of fullness in your stomach.

When your stomach is full after eating, stretch receptors in its walls send a signal to the vagus nerve, which tells your brain to stop eating because enough food has been consumed. One of the many reasons I recommend a diet based on high-fibre plant foods is because it fills you up so much more effectively than any other type of food, enabling the brain to receive the signal that you're full.

To use calories as a reference, imagine the difference between 400 calories of vegetables, olive oil and beef in your stomach. You would need to eat plenty of veggies to get 400 calories' worth (about six cups each of lettuce, aubergine and tomatoes), but they would really fill you up since they're so rich in water and fibre.

However, just under 3½ tablespoons of oil or just under a cup of sliced beef quickly add up to 400 calories, and without all the dietary fibre to tell your stomach's stretch receptors that you've eaten enough because animal protein contains no dietary fibre. It shows how important it is to fill up on veggies to help with weight management.

What your food cravings really mean

No matter how healthy and balanced your lifestyle is, almost everyone will face food cravings at some stage. But did you know that the type of foods you crave may tell you a lot about the essential nutrients that you could be lacking? Your body may be in need of various nutrients, which the brain interprets as cravings for certain foods. These are often sugary, salty, starchy or fatty snacks.

FULL OF FOOD, STARVED OF NUTRIENTS

Eating a diet that's high in refined carbs, processed foods and nutrient-depleted foods can often lead to food cravings, as your body struggles to get the wide array of nutrients it requires each day for normal and healthy function. These foods can cause extreme blood sugar fluctuations, which may really impact your mood and energy levels and trigger food cravings. While you may be eating a lot, your body can still be malnourished because it's not getting the nutrients it needs, so your brain tells you to keep on eating.

Being in touch with your body and your food cravings can make all the difference to your health and maintaining your ideal body weight. When a craving arises, it really helps to know why it's happening and what foods can ease without impacting your health or waistline.

ARE YOU WONDERING WHAT YOUR FOOD CRAVINGS ARE TELLING YOU?

Here's a handy guide to why you might crave certain foods and some healthy alternatives to choose.

1

CRAVING CHOCOLATE

This is often a sign that your body is lacking magnesium, which is nature's sedating hormone and essential for easing stress and anxiety, relaxing muscles, enabling energy production, building healthy bones and for normal heart function. Instead of reaching for a bar of chocolate, try eating raw nuts and seeds, leafy green veggies or one of my healthier chocolate treats, such as the fitness fudge brownies on page 237. Raw cacao powder is a super source of magnesium and antioxidants and banana is an excellent good mood food too.

2

CRAVING SWEETS

This may also be linked to magnesium deficiency. Try incorporating more nuts, seeds and leafy greens into your diet. Almonds and avocados are both good sources of magnesium, and my stress-soothing avocado smoothie on page 152 is rich in this essential mineral.

If my body needs a quick energy fix, I usually crave sweet fruits like banana, pineapple or grapes rather than refined sugar or stodgy carbs. I find them perfect for a pre-workout snack, as they provide clean-burning, instant energy.

But if I'm tired and craving a sugar hit, I eat a handful of raw almonds, pumpkin seeds and raisins sprinkled with cinnamon, which work together to help produce serotonin and lift my mood.

3

CRAVING SALTY FOODS

You need a small amount of chloride each day for healthy bodily function (about ¼ teaspoon), so cravings for salty foods may indicate that you need a little bit of salt to balance levels. In that case, I recommend using a pinch of Celtic sea salt or Himalayan pink rock salt rather than refined table salt, as they're both richer in minerals and more natural than processed salt.

But salt cravings can also be related to stress. When you're highly stressed or feeling under pressure, your adrenal glands produce excessive levels of cortisol. This stress hormone may cause you to crave high-fat, stodgy foods, including crisps and chips. Once again, stress management is essential.

Salty foods may cause you to look and feel a few pounds heavier, as they can dehydrate the body and encourage your kidneys to send out the signal to store water rather than excrete it. Avoiding salty foods or adding extra salt to foods, plus drinking plenty of water, can help to release water retention for leaner limbs and a flatter stomach.

4

CRAVING FATTY FOODS

According to a Harvard Medical School study, 'Once ingested, fat-filled foods seem to have a feedback effect that inhibits activity in the parts of the brain that produce and process stress and related emotions.' This means that many people could view fatty foods such as chips and cheese as comfort food, then crave them when they feel sad or stressed.

Cravings for these fatty foods may also indicate a lack of essential fats in your body, such as omega-3 and omega-6 fatty acids. To boost health and ease cravings for fat, try eating a handful of raw unsalted walnuts or adding a tablespoon of chia seeds, ground flaxseeds or hemp seeds to smoothies, porridge, soups and salads every day.

5

CRAVING FIZZY DRINKS

This may indicate a need for more calcium in your body, and Irish adults require 800mg of calcium per day. Calcium can be found in dark green leafy vegetables such as kale, broccoli and collard greens as well as in dried beans and legumes. Other good sources include tahini (sesame seed butter), dried figs, flaxseeds, chia seeds, calcium-fortified plant milks, oranges and almonds.

Many people associate dairy with calcium, but scientists from the prestigious US Harvard School of Public Health have stated, 'Calcium is important. But milk isn't the only, or even best, source.'

6

CRAVING TEA OR COFFEE

Many of us love a daily cup of tea or coffee, especially in the morning. But craving these hot drinks all day can indicate a deficiency of phosphorus in your system. Phosphorus is important for proper cell functioning, energy production, the regulation of calcium, and strong bones and teeth.

Some of the best plant-based sources of the mineral include almonds, pumpkin seeds, Brazil nuts, beans, mushrooms and sesame seeds.

7

CRAVING BREAD

Cravings for bread may happen when you're stressed or following a low-carb diet, but it may also be because your body requires more nitrogen. Nitrogen can be consumed in high-protein foods, including beans and legumes, nuts and seeds and quinoa, as well as animal-based protein if you're not eating a plant-based diet.

It's all about balance

One of the questions I'm asked most often by those interested in my lifestyle is whether I get cravings for 'unhealthy' foods. My honest response is that it does happen sometimes, but not very often, as I've learned how to balance my diet and ensure I'm getting all the nutrients I need. My body never thinks that it's being starved or deprived of essential nutrients. Also, I follow a plant-based diet because I really enjoy experimenting with the foods and flavours. It's definitely not a punishment!

I'm only human though and I do enjoy breaking 'the rules' from time to time. In my twenties there were times when I tried to be the absolute 'healthiest' version of myself. And you know what? I wasn't very happy or healthy doing it, because I would feel immense guilt for missing workouts or eating something I had told myself I shouldn't. Life is for living to the full, enjoying fun times with friends and treating yourself every so often.

Be kind to yourself, avoid crash diets, eat
sensibly as much as possible and never feel
guilty for enjoying your life and treating
yourself. But for the best quality of life,
I believe it's important to eat and drink
moderately and to strike a sustainable
balance between health, fitness and fun
to help you feel your very best. Be good
80% of the time and enjoy yourself for the
remaining 20%.

It's not about being perfect all the time.
It's about balance and progress.

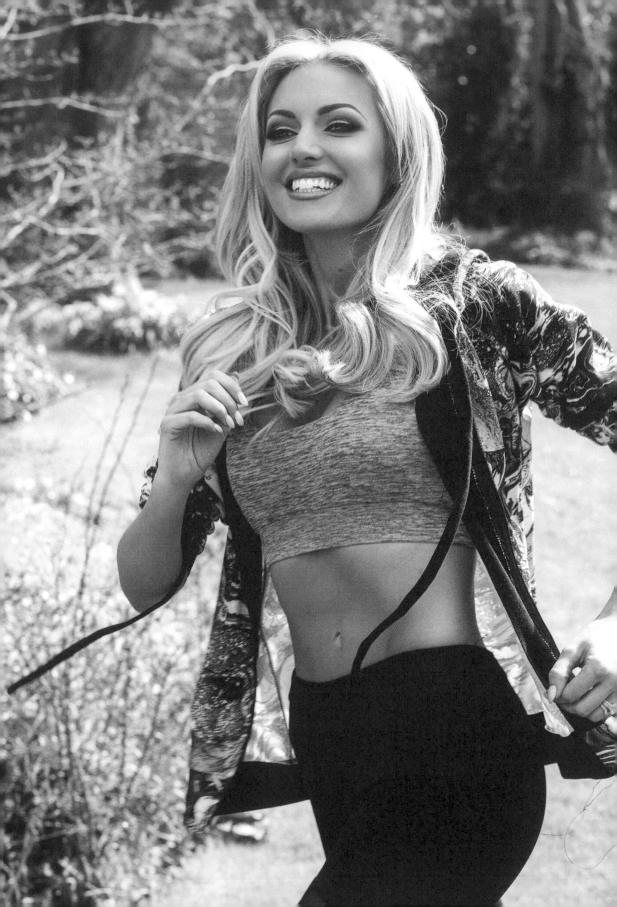

PART 4

MIND, BODY AND SOUL

"To keep the body in good health is a duty ...
otherwise we shall not be able
to keep our mind strong and clear."

BUDDHA

The brain and gut mood connection

Did you know that the health of your digestive system may affect your mood? There is a complex network of neurons lining your gut that's so detailed and extensive, it's been nicknamed the 'second brain'.

This 'second brain' is technically known as the enteric nervous system and consists of sheaths of neurons embedded in the walls of your digestive tract. It contains around 100 million neurons, which is even more than in either the spinal cord or the peripheral nervous system. This allows the complicated digestive process to be fully completed without involving the actual brain too much.

This incredible network of nerves may also have a large influence on your emotional well-being, and not just feeling butterflies in your stomach when you're nervous or excited. The enteric nervous system uses more than 30 neurotransmitters, just like the brain, and it's estimated that at least 90% of the body's serotonin is actually found in the gut.

It's important to look after your digestive health to encourage efficient digestion and a bloat-free stomach as well as a good mood. You can do this by eating plenty of high-fibre plant foods, taking probiotics regularly to populate your gut with 'friendly' bacteria, eating fermented foods for their probiotic qualities, avoiding foods that may irritate or inflame your gut, and consuming 'good mood foods' with every meal and snack.

GOOD MOOD FOOD

Certain foods encourage your body and brain to produce the neurotransmitters and hormones that can help to make you feel happy, calm and positive and encourage restful sleep. Normal and healthy levels of serotonin even assist in preventing cravings for sugary, fatty and stodgy foods, thus ensuring that you're eating plenty of good mood foods each day can really help to keep your health and fitness on track.

These are the best types of good mood food.

1

PROTEIN

If you don't eat enough protein, your moods may suffer and you could find it difficult to feel positive, happy, optimistic and calm. Instead, feelings of anxiety, depression and low self-esteem may creep in, along with unhealthy food cravings.

The various neurotransmitters that help you to feel cheerful are formed from the amino acids in foods, especially those richer in protein. Whether or not you eat meat, poultry, fish and eggs, I would encourage you to eat some protein foods with every meal or snack. The protein foods that contain the serotonin precursor, tryptophan, are especially important for boosting your mood. I feel the benefits from eating lentils, chickpeas, hummus, quinoa, almonds, walnuts, chia seeds, hemp seeds, nutritional yeast and adding a plant-based protein powder to smoothies and smoothie bowls. All those foods are a complete source of essential amino acids, especially tryptophan, and feature in many of my *Eat Yourself Fit* recipes.

2

FAT

Fat is incredibly important, especially for women, as it's needed for producing and regulating your hormones. The human brain contains up to 60% fat and requires a consistent stream of healthy fats to keep it working optimally, but you need to feed it regularly with the right type of fatty foods.

OMEGA-3 FAT

Omega-3 fat is the most important type for your brain and body. It nourishes every single body cell to keep them strong and supple, it helps your complexion to stay fresh and youthful, it keeps joints lubricated and healthy, and the more of it you eat, the better your mood can become.

This is because it has been shown to quickly increase a natural and potent antidepressant brain chemical called dopamine by up to 40%, boosting alertness, focus and a good mood.

Omega-3 fats are found in chia seeds, hemp seeds, flaxseeds and flax oil, walnuts, chlorella and spirulina and in oily fish, including wild salmon, sardines and mackerel. I often supplement with a plant-based micro-algae omega-3 capsule, which I find especially useful in winter, when my skin feels drier. If you suffer with dry skin and hair, low moods or anxiety, then you may very well benefit from a good-quality omega-3 supplement.

OMEGA-6 FAT

It's best to limit foods higher in omega-6 fats, which include margarine, vegetable oils, commercial salad dressings, mayonnaise, deep-fried foods, chips, crisps, sausages, bacon, salami, ham, pork chops, beef and certain eggs.

Some nuts are higher in omega-6 fats, including almonds, peanuts, pecans and pumpkin seeds, but as they have numerous other health benefits, I don't suggest consciously limiting or avoiding them. Instead, try to balance them well with chia, hemp, flaxseeds and walnuts.

OILS

I generally recommend using pure oils of any type sparingly, as they are considered a processed food devoid of fibre and are high in calories. But pure, cold-pressed extra virgin olive oil is the best option for salads and when used in moderation. Avoid using it for cooking, though, as it's unstable at high temperatures.

Olive oil is a better oil than other vegetable oils for dips and salads because it's high in omega-9 fats, with little omega-6 fats, so it doesn't go rancid as easily. Though relatively low in omega-3s, the omega-9s in olive oil support the omega-3s and encourage the antidepressant activities of serotonin in the brain.

SATURATED FAT

Sat fats haven't enjoyed the best reputation over the years, and many people wouldn't associate them with good health and a happy mood. But unsweetened dried coconut, coconut oil and coconut milk are my favourite types of saturated fat to enjoy regularly, and they appear in plenty of my recipes too.

Coconut boasts incredible antibacterial and antifungal properties and remains stable at high temperatures, which is why its oil works so well in cooking. However, coconut oil is still best used sparingly if you're trying to lose some body fat, as there are about 120 calories per tablespoon, which can quickly add up if you use it regularly.

3

VEGETABLES AND FRUIT

They're bright, colourful, juicy and energising! Veggies and fruit are packed with vitamins, minerals, fibre, antioxidants and phytonutrients for protecting your cells and boosting your mood. Think of them as the essential partner to the good mood proteins and fats, which contribute the nutrients that your brain needs the most. Vegetables also boost energy without raising your blood sugar levels.

Try to start your day with a big smoothie packed with leafy greens and a little fruit, then include plenty of raw, lightly steamed or baked veggies with your lunch, evening meal and even your snacks. For so long, animal protein has been the main focus of meals – I believe it's time to prioritise vegetables for their incredible mood benefits and protection against a wide range of modern lifestyle diseases.

Their rich content of B vitamins, the antioxidant vitamins A, C and E, beta-carotene, magnesium and potassium help to boost energy levels, support healthy blood pressure, build younger-looking skin and strengthen your immune system. Aim to eat at least seven to nine servings of colourful fruit and vegetables each day.

Fruit tends to be easy to digest for most people. Bananas are a particularly good source of vitamin B6, which is needed to produce serotonin. All fruit is rich in the antioxidants that protect the cell membranes in your brain, supporting neurotransmitter activity.

The main sugar in fruit is fructose, which is slower to convert into glucose than regular refined sugar. As it's also rich in fibre, fruit doesn't tend to cause fluctuations in blood sugar levels for most people. Fruit is best eaten on an empty stomach as a snack or before a meal.

Organic produce is ideal when it's available, but make sure you rinse all fresh fruit and veg well before eating them and avoid overcooking to preserve their nutrients. Lightly steamed or sautéed vegetables work well for most people.

Starchy vegetables such as butternut squash and sweet potato, beans and legumes, and ancient grains including quinoa, buckwheat and millet are nutritious and mood-boosting foods too. The starchier veggies tend to be easy to digest and high in potassium and beta-carotene, while beans, legumes and grains are generally rich in blood sugar-stabilising protein and fibre. These will need to be rinsed well and even soaked prior to cooking from dry.

BAD MOOD FOOD

The typical Western diet tends to be heavy in nutrient-depleted and low-fibre processed foods. Many people skip meals, especially breakfast, and don't eat enough vegetables or omega-3 fat, while others may be low in essential vitamins and minerals and eat too many foods high in empty calories.

So what does that mean for your mood? Between the nutrient-depleted foods you do eat and the good mood foods that you don't eat, it's the perfect recipe for a mood disaster. If you survive on caffeine, sugar, sweet or diet fizzy drinks, biscuits, cereal, chocolate or bread to pull you through your day, then you're not only causing potential long-term damage to your body weight and metabolism, you're also setting yourself up for low moods.

Here are the worst foods for your mood.

1

REFINED SUGAR AND WHITE FLOUR

This sugar–starch terrible twosome crops up in everything from pastries to biscuits, cakes, breads, crackers, packaged cereals and a wide range of baked goods, while sugar is found in a vast array of sweet and savoury food, from sweets and fizzy drinks to yogurts, breads, jams, soups, sauces and savoury condiments.

Sugar is one of the world's most addictive substances, described by many experts as the cocaine of the culinary world. It can have a devastating effect on your health, waistline, emotions and mood. The wide availability of sugar and its addictive nature makes you especially vulnerable, and millions of people are hooked on sugar.

When paired with white flour, sugar becomes even more of a problem for your health and waistline. Just like sweets, white breads and sweetened cereals are converted into glucose, which raises blood sugar dramatically in a very short space of time. This triggers the release of insulin, which stores excess glucose as body fat, especially around a woman's stomach, hips, thighs and upper arms, and a man's abdominal region.

Due to the extraction process that these foods undergo, their beneficial fibre, vitamins and minerals are almost completely removed, leaving a concentrated substance so potent that it can force your brain to release its feel-good neurotransmitters. You feel temporarily uplifted and happy when you eat the starch and sugar combo, until the positive chemicals are depleted and you crave another hit to achieve a brief boost to your mood, and the addictive cycle continues.

2
WHEAT

Millions of people around the world eat a diet based on wheat products containing gluten. Many don't notice any issues with it, as not everybody is affected by wheat, rye and barley. But for some people, these grains can have a negative effect on their body, digestive system, energy levels and mood.

Those diagnosed with coeliac disease must avoid all gluten products, and plenty of others either feel better by omitting it or notice digestive difficulties, bloating and even inflammatory conditions arise from eating it. I try to avoid gluten as I discovered that it may trigger acne breakouts as well as stomach cramps, bloating and low energy because I struggle to digest it. Rye and barley contain less gluten than wheat, but if you're sensitive to gluten, then they're best avoided. Oats are a naturally gluten-free grain but may become cross-contaminated in

the transport and storage process, so that's why I recommend certified gluten-free oats. Pseudo-grains including quinoa, millet and amaranth, as well as rice and corn pasta, can be a huge help to those avoiding gluten. There are also plenty of gluten-free alternatives to bread, biscuits, muffins and cakes available in most shops and supermarkets now, and all the recipes in this book are gluten-free.

3
VEGETABLE OILS AND MARGARINE

This list of bad mood fats includes corn oil, soy oil, canola oil, safflower oil, sunflower oil, peanut oil, sesame oil, cottonseed oil and wheat germ oil. They're the oils used in a vast amount of baked goods, packaged meals, salad dressings, sauces and mayonnaise.

My reason for listing them in this category is because of their unstable nature, as they can become rancid quickly. Much like an apple that turns brown when exposed to the air, these oils often become oxidised from heat and light, and consuming may cause damage to your body cells. By eating them, you're exposing your body to a potentially unstable and damaging substance, and fat-rich brain tissue is especially vulnerable to the effects.

Furthermore, most of these vegetable oils are rich in omega-6 fats. While it's an essential fat that humans require in small amounts regularly, it's also a type of fat that can encourage inflammation in your cells and tissues. A little inflammation is perfectly normal and is an important part of your immune system's response, but including too many omega-6 fats in your regular diet may interfere with the neuro-transmitter function in your brain cells.

Many animal protein foods, including poultry, meat and fish, are raised on omega-6 grains rather than fresh grass and algae, which are lower in omega-6 and high in omega-3. That is why I recommend you source high-quality organic grass-fed meats, wild fish and flax-fed poultry and eggs if you choose to consume animal products.

Trans fats can be damaging to your mood because they may prevent your brain from properly utilising protective omega-3 fats, allowing omega-6 fats to dominate.

4

SOY PRODUCTS

Marketed as the ideal plant protein source, soy has pervaded the food industry over the past few decades. Those selling it refer to the longevity of Asian populations, who are known for eating soy products. But not all soy is made equal, and it remains a controversial topic. Limited amounts of soy sauce are used as a condiment and, similarly, small amounts of tofu in miso soup.

Some studies do show that two isoflavones found in soy, called genistein and daidzein, may be protective against many types of cancer. This is because they have properties that mimic your own oestrogen. The fibre in soy can improve your digestive health.

However, other studies show that 'phytoestrogens' such as these may also increase the risk for hormone-dependent cancers including breast and ovarian cancer. A 2007 report in a peer-reviewed journal of the American Cancer Society found that soy products may stimulate breast cancer cell growth in women before they hit menopause, but can protect against it in post-menopausal women.

Rather worryingly, much of the Western world's soy has been genetically engineered, which can dramatically change the inter-action of nutrients in various foods. They can have significantly fewer minerals required for your nervous system develop-ment and more compounds that may spark food allergies and sensitivities. Many people report an allergy to soy, and it's in the top 10 most allergenic foods in America.

SOY AND YOUR THYROID

Your thyroid is the delicate butterfly gland in front of your windpipe, which controls the metabolism of every cell in your body. Soybeans contain goitrogens, which are substances that can actually block your thyroid hormones from being made. As their name suggests, this can lead to goitre, a swelling of the neck that indicates an enlarged thyroid gland. The main goitrogens in soy are their isoflavones, which research has found to depress the function of your thyroid and slow down your entire metabolism. This may lead to weight gain, dry skin and other health concerns. There is an abundance of research suggesting that soy isoflavones are toxic to thyroid tissue and oestrogen-related tissues.

So what can you do to benefit most from soy products? You can certainly enjoy it in its fermented form. This disbands the inhibitors in soy and makes it much more easy for your body to process and without the risks I've mentioned. Some great options include miso soup, tempeh and tamari sauce, which is similar in taste to soy sauce but is gluten free.

Low serotonin and sugar cravings

Serotonin is one of your most important brain neurotransmitters for a positive mental attitude and better-quality sleep. Up to 90% of the chemical is actually produced in your digestive tract, but low levels in your brain may lead to irritability, lowered motivation, depression, poor sleep and powerful cravings for sugary and stodgy comfort foods.

According to scientific research, the levels of serotonin in your brain may have a big influence on your eating choices. Tryptophan is the essential amino acid that produces serotonin, with the help of co-factors including vitamin B6 and zinc.

Pioneering research conducted at the Massachusetts Institute of Technology discovered that when humans are fed diets specially formulated to be deficient in tryptophan, their appetite dramatically increases, which leads to binge-eating carbs and refined sugar. The low tryptophan diet can cause low brain serotonin, which the brain interprets as a starvation state, and then powerfully stimulates appetite control hormones.

This type of stimulation makes you crave carbs over every other type of food because a high-carbohydrate meal raises insulin, which helps deliver tryptophan to the brain quickly, enabling serotonin to be formed. Therefore, low serotonin levels trigger carbohydrate cravings and may play a significant part in the progression of weight gain.

SUPPORT YOUR SEROTONIN

If you're trying to lose a few pounds of body fat or maintain your current weight, then it's important to look after your serotonin levels every day to help prevent cravings and food binges.

1

Eat a diet sufficient in protein and especially tryptophan-rich foods, such as almonds, almond milk, almond butter, pumpkin seeds, sunflower seeds, cashews and walnuts, which all contain over 50 milligrams of tryptophan in a quarter of a cup. Legumes such as lentils, beans and peas provide around 180 milligrams per cup.

2

Eat some protein with every meal and snack throughout the day to help keep blood sugar levels stable and provide tryptophan to boost serotonin. A high-quality protein powder can also be helpful in boosting protein and tryptophan levels, and I use one in plenty of my recipes.

3

Exercise regularly to boost your feel-good endorphins and serotonin levels and to oxygenate your body and brain. Physical activity also helps to burn body fat and encourage healthy food choices.

4

Avoid stimulants that many lower serotonin levels, particularly recreational drugs and excessive alcohol. The high that they provide can be followed by lowered serotonin, which may last a few days as your brain and body recover and rebalance.

5

Get sufficient sleep. Research consistently links insufficient sleep with low brain serotonin levels, which may trigger cravings for sugary and stodgy snacks.

6

Track the pattern of what triggers food cravings and have a back-up plan in place. For many people, cravings for sugary, salty and fatty foods can arise in the evening time, particularly on winter nights. Try one of the many *Eat Yourself Fit* sweet treats and creamy smoothies to satisfy a sweet tooth.

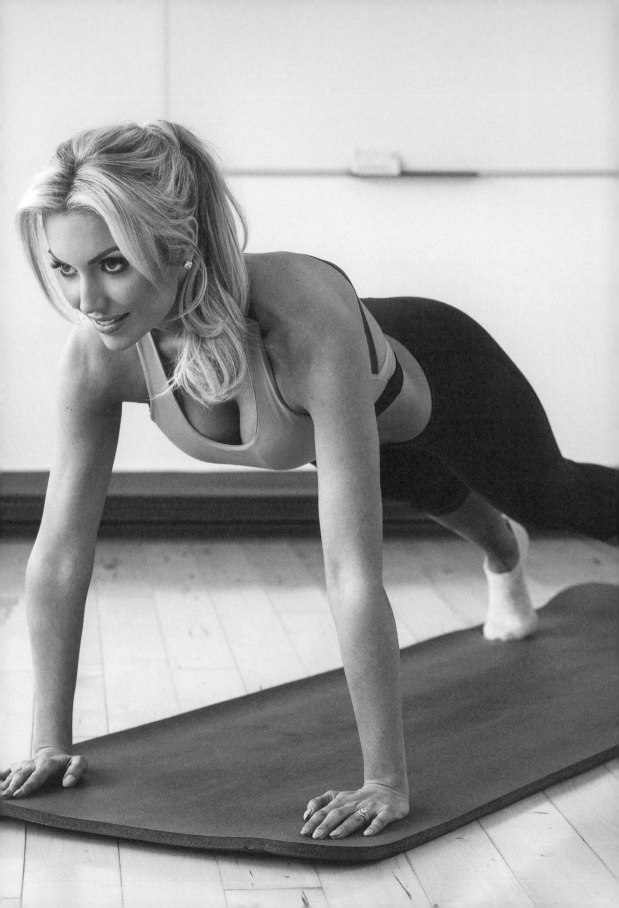

PMS

The normal fluctuations in a woman's hormones each month can greatly affect your mood, and there's a close connection between your reproductive hormones and the various neurotransmitters you need to support a good mood.

It's estimated that three out of every four women experience pre-menstrual syndrome (PMS) to some extent, with symptoms including irritability, depression, crying spells, increased hunger, food cravings, headache, fluid retention, bloating and breast tenderness. Generally women will experience only a few of these symptoms, which can begin up to 14 days before a woman's period and typically go away when it starts.

Interactions between your hormones and neurotransmitters (brain chemicals), plus stress and poor diet and food choices, are generally thought to trigger or worsen PMS. But there are certain steps you can take to ease the symptoms and boost your feel-good endorphins.

1

EAT REGULAR MEALS AND SNACKS

Eating a small meal or snack every three to four hours really helps to keep blood sugar levels stable and boost energy levels throughout the day. It also stabilises your mood and helps to keep PMS-induced irritability at bay. Stopping every few hours to focus on how you feel and to eat something if you notice a drop in energy can help to keep emotions stable.

The best type of meal or snack to lift a PMS mood contains protein, fibre and healthy fats. Some of my favourites include veggie sticks with hummus, oatcakes with guacamole and fresh apple wedges or apple crisps with almond butter (see the recipe on page 233).

2

EAT MAGNESIUM-RICH FOODS

Magnesium is known as nature's sedating nutrient for good reason, as it helps to calm a stressed-out nervous system, relax your muscles, regulate blood pressure, heart rate and blood sugar levels, maintain nerve function and ease PMS.

Ever wonder why some women crave chocolate just before their period? Ounce for ounce, dark chocolate contains more magnesium than any other type of food. It's an important mineral that research shows many adults may be deficient in. Everybody benefits from a magnesium-rich diet, but magnesium levels may fluctuate throughout a woman's cycle, with higher levels of oestrogen or progesterone leading to lowered magnesium levels. A magnesium-rich diet can help relieve PMS-related symptoms, such as headaches, bloating, low blood sugar, dizziness, fluid retention and sugar cravings.

Chocolate in its raw and unprocessed form helps the most. The raw cacao powder that I use to create many of my desserts and sweet treats is loaded with essential minerals, including calcium, sulphur, zinc, iron, copper, potassium and manganese. It's also full of antioxidant flavonoids to protect your cells from damage, a range of the B vitamins, protein and fibre.

Apart from chocolate, good food sources of magnesium include leafy green vegetables, almonds, cashews, avocado, sunflower seeds, pumpkin seeds and buckwheat.

3

INDULGE IN CHOCOLATE

Another key reason why women may crave chocolate at a certain time of the month is because levels of serotonin may decrease along with oestrogen and progesterone to trigger the start of your period. Without sufficient serotonin, you may crave sugary foods or stodgy carbs to quickly and naturally boost levels back up again.

Commercial chocolate generally isn't a great option because it tends to be full of refined sugar, so I designed my SOS chocolate bark on page 242 to come to the rescue when only chocolate will do. It's naturally sweetened to help boost serotonin without the subsequent energy crash that can happen with regular refined sugar.

4

EAT FOODS RICH IN B VITAMINS

B vitamins, including thiamine (B1), riboflavin (B2), B3, B5, B6 and folic acid, are found in a large range of foods, including veggies, oats, quinoa, nuts, seeds, lentils and beans.

They're essential for many biochemical reactions in your body, including energy production. As a water-soluble vitamin, you must eat enough in your food each day, and real food is generally a better idea than relying on supplements.

Vitamins B1 and B2 can be important for easing PMS. According to a US study published in the online edition of *The American Journal of Clinical Nutrition*, women with higher intakes of them in their diet had far fewer PMS symptoms.

5

PRIORITISE OMEGA-3 FATS

Increasing your dietary intake of omega-3 fats can be effective in reducing PMS symptoms. According to the peer-reviewed journal *Complementary Therapies in Medicine*, omega-3 fats can help to lessen feelings of depression, nervousness, anxiety and lack of concentration. They may also reduce bloating, headache and breast tenderness due to their powerful anti-inflammatory properties.

Many people eating the typical Western diet consume too many omega-6 and omega-9 fats from vegetable oils, fried foods and animal protein foods, but not enough omega-3 fats. This may impact PMS, so rebalancing the fatty acids in your system is thought to offer relief.

Beauty sleep

As one of the most important physiological functions, sleep is of the highest value to your health, fitness and emotional well-being. Adults need at least seven to eight hours of snooze time per night, but many people fall short of that for a variety of reasons. Various chemicals and compounds found in foods and drinks can also have a powerful effect on your sleeping patterns.

You need sleep to help regulate your appetite hormones, with studies showing that not getting sufficient shut-eye may increase your daily calorie intake by up to 20%. This could cause weight gain in the long term.

NUTRIENTS FOR SLEEP

The right balance of nutrients is needed by your body to keep it working optimally throughout the night, as it heals the day's cellular damage and resets your system.

Foods naturally rich in calcium and magnesium are good for encouraging sleep, as they help to relax your muscles. Try eating foods rich in both nutrients with your evening meal. Good sources include leafy green vegetables, broccoli, almonds, chickpeas, dried figs, cashews, sesame seeds, tahini, quinoa and kidney beans.

If you have trouble getting a decent night's sleep, aim to avoid biscuits, chocolate, sweets and other refined sugar foods close to bedtime. They can raise your blood sugar levels, then the insulin response can cause a sudden dip in blood glucose. Your body responds by sending out a wave of adrenaline, which may wake you up with a sudden jolt in the middle of the night.

MELATONIN, YOUR SLEEP HORMONE

Do you ever feel increasingly sleepy earlier in the evenings as winter approaches? Your levels of the sleep hormone, melatonin, rise steadily as darkness falls each night.

Produced by the pineal gland in your brain, melatonin is made in particularly large quantities when you are young. As well as regulating your snooze patterns, melatonin is an extremely powerful antioxidant and even more effective than the A, C and E vitamins for neutralising the free radicals that can damage and age your cells prematurely. It's also been shown to support your immune system.

When you wake up in the morning and it's already daylight, the light hitting your retina triggers neurological signals that cause melatonin production to halt. That's why it can be difficult to get out of bed when the alarm clock goes off on dark mornings!

Darkness and light are two key triggers for melatonin production, but various dietary and lifestyle factors can help to regulate your melatonin to ensure you get deep, good-quality sleep and wake up feeling refreshed.

Eating meals and snacks at regular intervals and not going too many hours without food will help to regulate your body's routine and its melatonin levels. Eating heavy meals too late in the evening may interrupt your internal chemistry and affect sleep.

Get used to going to bed at a similar time each night and waking up at the same time each morning, and avoid napping during the day if you can. This will aid in regulating your circadian rhythm and cortisol production, which should be at its peak first thing in the morning to help kick start your day.

REDUCE CAFFEINE

If you have trouble settling down or sleeping, then it can really help to limit tea, coffee, excess chocolate, nicotine, caffeinated soft drinks and energy drinks, as caffeine remains in your system for up to 24 hours and keeps you feeling alert. Chamomile tea has a subtle sedative effect and is a natural relaxant before bed.

AVOID TYRAMINE FOODS

Foods containing the amino acid tyramine, including bacon, ham, sausage, chocolate, sugar, cheese and wine, are also best avoided close to bedtime as they have been shown to stimulate norepinephrine in your brain, which can act as a stimulant and keep you awake.

EXERCISE EARLIER IN THE DAY

Intense exercise too close to bedtime may actually delay melatonin production, energise you and keep you from getting to sleep. A good workout is a brilliant way to ensure you get a good night's sleep, but it's best done earlier in the day if possible. This means that you will feel full of energy for the day and encourage a natural balance of melatonin in your system.

TRYPTOPHAN FOODS

The amino acid tryptophan is needed along with vitamins B6, B12, folic acid and zinc to build serotonin and melatonin. A diet lacking any of these nutrients, or one that's low in overall protein, may cause you sleep problems.

Eating a tryptophan-rich snack one or two hours before bedtime can really help to produce melatonin for peaceful sleep. Good options include a handful of raw nuts and blueberries, chopped apple with a teaspoon of hazelnut butter, sliced banana with a sprinkle of pumpkin and sunflower seeds or a cup of warm unsweetened almond milk with a pinch of cinnamon.

A positive mental attitude

Your body and brain are deeply interlinked. Harmony must be promoted throughout both, because a positive mental attitude as you grow and develop through life is very much at the foundation of vitality. When you're feeling positive, strong, happy and resilient, you glow with health and contentment.

Of course, you can go through life eating and drinking what you please and avoiding exercise, but this may eventually start to break down your health and resilience to disease. Taking the time to look after the body that works so hard to keep you alive and well every single day hugely improves your quality of life, energy levels, long-term wellness, self-confidence and the love and time that you can give to your friends and family.

Just like your physical fitness, a positive mental attitude takes ongoing work and attention to stay healthy. Working hard to remain full of positivity and optimism throughout your life is so important and there is an ever-increasing body of scientific evidence that your regular thoughts, emotions and self-image very much contribute to your health and quality of life.

You can't control much of what life throws at you and all of us will face our own challenges, but what you *can* control is how you respond to these challenges and your ongoing attitude. It's how you respond to the many difficulties that you face that moulds your character and quality of life.

The failures, losses, broken hearts, hardships and sadness most of us will face frequently end up nourishing your happiness, achievements and empathy for others. Adopting a positive attitude will ensure that you're happier, healthier and more successful in all areas of life. Don't forget that like attracts like. Make yourself a magnet for happiness, joy, good health and success. I find that meditation, deep breathing and remembering to be grateful for all that makes you happy in life can really help to encourage a calm, positive mindset.

Setting positive goals is absolutely essential for creating an optimistic attitude and building your self-confidence. You must word your statement of intent to achieve these goals in positive language, and it can also be applied to getting healthy and fit: 'I love to eat healthy fruit and vegetables and exercise every day' is a much more positive statement than telling yourself 'I must not eat sugar, junk food or bread and I am not allowed to skip the gym'. Of course you're going to rebel against that. I know I would!

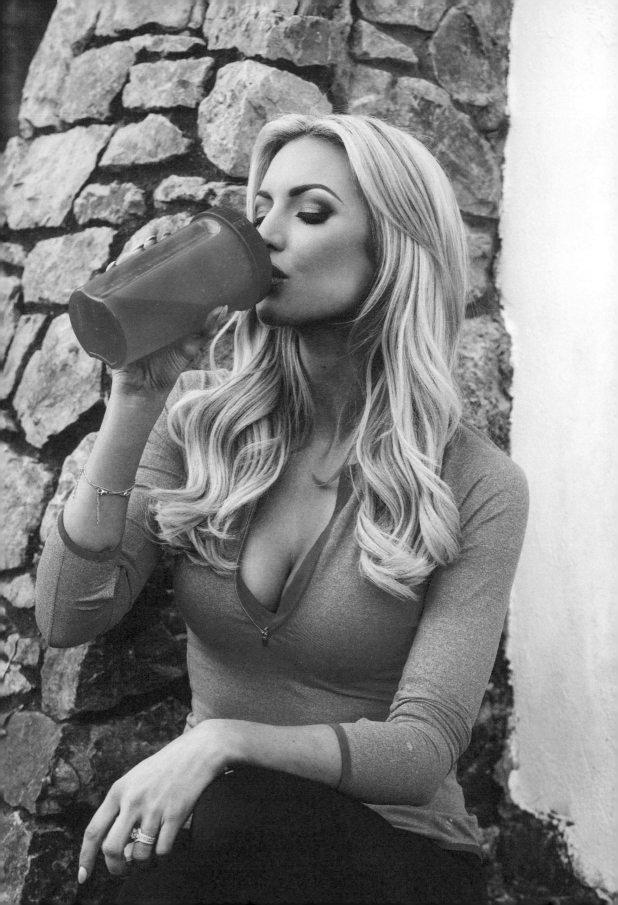

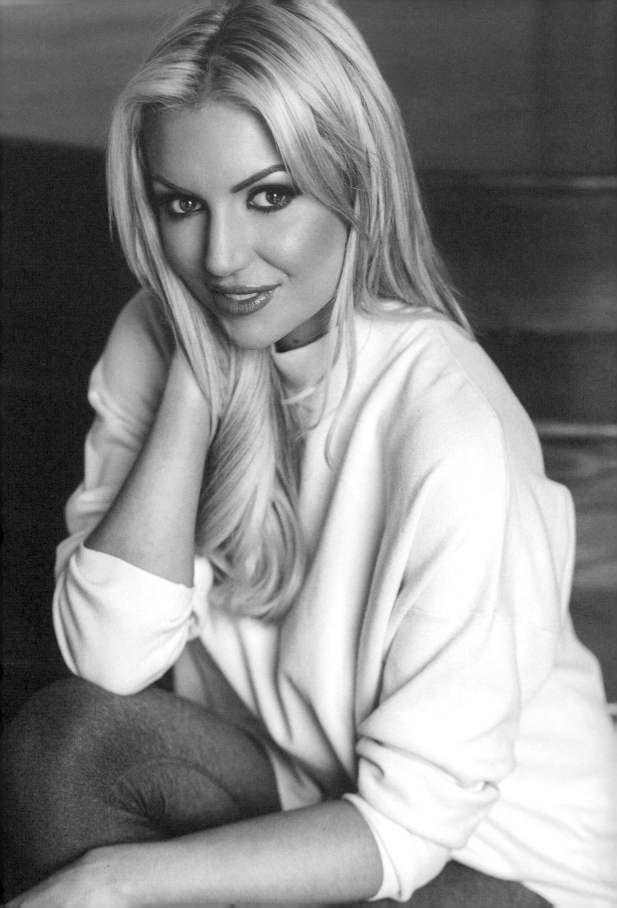

PART 5

THE *EAT YOURSELF FIT* ULTIMATE BODY PLAN

This plan is all about putting the information in the previous chapters into practice using the *Eat Yourself Fit* recipes. It's one thing having the knowledge, but you need to be able to make it work for you when life is busy and to see a discernible difference in your body, fitness, energy levels and overall health.

This seven-day sample food plan is one that I closely follow whenever I want to tighten and tone up my body, flatten my stomach and reduce any bloating ahead of a holiday, photo shoot or important event. You may want to follow it for just one week or longer, but it's not meant to be a quick-fix crash diet, so it's perfectly okay to take your time to ease into it if that's what you need. Remember, progress, not perfection.

The plan will work most effectively if you follow my advice closely, but don't worry if you have a bad day or struggle to resist other temptations. Health is not built nor destroyed in 24 hours, so you can get back on track the following day. Healthy eating shouldn't be viewed as a punishment!

I have carefully designed an approximately 1,300 daily calorie plan packed with protein- and fibre-rich whole foods to help lower insulin levels and encourage maximum fat burning. I use only complex carbs in my meals and snacks to help maintain steady blood sugar levels, so your body will receive the full set of vitamins, minerals, essential fats and amino acids while maintaining a calorie deficit to help trigger body fat loss if that is your goal.

To make this plan work even harder for you, I advise that you download the cronometer.com or MyFitnessPal app or access either website on a computer. It will ask you to log in your height, weight and activity levels to accurately determine your own individual calorie needs, so you may need to add more food to my plan or slightly less, depending on your body, exercise regime and personal goals.

Calorie needs can vary greatly, so if you have any concerns you should consult an expert before embarking on the fitness plan.

For the plan to work effectively, it's really important that you pay attention to portion sizes, try to stop eating before you feel really full and don't eat a large meal too close to bedtime. Even with some healthy foods, you need to watch how much you're eating to avoid taking in more energy than your body can use. As I have explained, nutrient-dense rather than calorie-dense foods should be forming the bulk of your diet. Filling up on oil-free green salads and light soups will make a big difference. It's also best to avoid fruit juices, full-fat milky coffees and fizzy drinks, as liquid calories can quickly add up.

If you work out regularly, my advice is to supplement with a good-quality protein powder after a weights or resistance workout to begin the process of muscle recovery and repair. I love protein smoothies to help deliver the nutrients quickly within that 45-minute post-training window. After a cardio or flexibility workout, aim to eat real food, such as a chopped apple with almond butter or one of the many *Eat Yourself Fit* healthy meals and snacks.

Try to drink a large glass of green smoothie or juice each morning for all the energy and skin-boosting benefits from the rich quantities of chlorophyll in the leafy greens.

You will find a full suggested shopping list on my website, www.RosannaDavisonNutrition.com.

Supplements

The supplements industry is huge, but high-quality real food is so much more beneficial than synthetic supplements, as nature has cleverly designed foods to deliver the nutrients that your body needs in the correct proportions. If unsure, consult a qualified health professional before beginning a course of supplements, as certain nutrients can interact with various medications and cause a risk to your health. However, if you're not managing to eat as well as you could or if you're trying to lose weight, then a quality multivitamin can offer valuable health protection by preventing a nutrient deficiency.

A well-planned whole food plant-based diet will give you all you need, and generally even more than those eating a typical Western diet, as the foods are full of vitamins, minerals, protective antioxidants, amino acids and fibre.

VITAMIN B12

Vitamin B12 is essential for the protection and growth of your nervous system. One of the only vitamins you need to supplement on a plant-based diet is B12, as it's found almost entirely in animal protein foods. B12 can be found in fortified plant milks, nutritional yeast and some sea vegetables, but my advice is to supplement B12 on a plant-based diet. The Irish recommended dietary allowance for adults is 3 micrograms per day and 4 micrograms during pregnancy.

I use a daily spray under my tongue of methylcobalamin, which is directly absorbed into the bloodstream.

VITAMIN D

Vitamin D deficiency can be a problem in colder climates. As a fat-soluble vitamin, it acts as both a vitamin and a hormone and is important for absorbing calcium and phosphorus. Vitamin D is therefore crucial for healthy bones and teeth, plus normal growth, strong muscles and a healthy heart. It boosts your immune system and thyroid function for a healthy metabolism too.

There are different types of vitamin D, but vitamin D3 (cholecalciferol) is made in the skin when you're in sunlight. As the most active form, it's the type that you need to supplement. Just 15 minutes in adequate sunlight three times a week ensures that you'll get enough vitamin D, but in the more northern European countries, the sunlight is not adequate enough between November and March for us to make vitamin D3 naturally. Supplementing is important for supporting your immunity and research even suggests it may help prevent depression.

Some plant foods contain vitamin D, such as oatmeal, dandelion greens, shiitake and chanterelle mushrooms, sweet potatoes and parsley. Plant milks like coconut and almond are usually fortified with it. I strongly recommend taking a daily vitamin D3 supplement and avoiding too much sun exposure due to the damage and ageing that UV light can do to your skin.

PROBIOTICS

I have already explained the importance of probiotics for digestive health, immune system support, preventing a bloated stomach and proper absorption of nutrients. There are plenty of different brands available, but I find the Udo's Choice Super 8 Probiotics work very well. The capsules need to be refrigerated and are best taken after your evening meal.

TRYPTOPHAN SNACK

For those who would like to improve their quality of sleep, I have suggested an optional evening snack rich in tryptophan to be eaten one to two hours before bed. This helps to stimulate the production of melatonin to promote restful sleep.

OMEGA-3 FATS

Sprinkle a couple tablespoons of ground raw flaxseeds onto soups, salads, smoothies or breakfasts each day to get plenty of skin-smoothing omega-3 fats. However, if you struggle with dry skin, dandruff or painful PMS, then it can be worth taking a good omega-3 supplement. I like the Nordic Naturals Algae Omega-3 daily capsules.

MONDAY

(1,321 CALORIES)

BREAKFAST (477 CALORIES)
Glass of warm water with fresh lemon juice
Green goddess smoothie plus (page 133)
Creamy chia pudding with raspberry coulis (page 110)

SNACK (104 CALORIES)
15 raw unsalted almonds

LUNCH (204 CALORIES)
Carrot noodle salad with ginger-miso dressing (page 168)

SNACK (212 CALORIES)
Blue warrior recovery shake (page 136)

DINNER (286 CALORIES)
Creamy mushroom and quinoa stroganoff (page 178)

TRYPTOPHAN SNACK (38 CALORIES)
250ml warm unsweetened almond milk with a pinch of cinnamon and a few drops of liquid stevia to sweeten (optional)

TUESDAY

(1,300 CALORIES)

BREAKFAST (209 CALORIES)

Glass of warm water with fresh lemon juice

Roast Portobello mushrooms stuffed with chilli-lime guacamole (page 129)

SNACK (197 CALORIES)

Lean green body booster (page 138)

LUNCH (305 CALORIES)

Carrot, coconut and red lentil soup (page 160)

Large green salad dressed with balsamic vinegar and lemon juice

SNACK (165 CALORIES)

1 sliced apple with 1 teaspoon almond butter

70g blueberries (about ½ cup)

DINNER (255 CALORIES)

Avocado, lemon and basil pesto courgetti (page 188)

TRYPTOPHAN SNACK (169 CALORIES)

1 banana mashed with cinnamon and 2 teaspoons raw nut or seed butter (no added sugar or palm oil)

WEDNESDAY

(1,266 CALORIES)

BREAKFAST (339 CALORIES)

Glass of warm water with fresh lemon juice

Glass of green goddess juice (page 134)

Creamy millet power porridge (page 100)

SNACK (106 CALORIES)

125g fresh blueberries or raspberries

10 raw unsalted almonds

LUNCH (140 CALORIES)

Lean green soup (page 159)

Skinny cauliflower tabbouleh with toasted sesame seeds (page 163)

SNACK (258 CALORIES)

Spicy roast chickpea bites (page 224)

DINNER (291 CALORIES)

Coconut curried quinoa with cheesy roast cauliflower (page 201)

TRYPTOPHAN SNACK (132 CALORIES)

Spiced apple crisps with 1 teaspoon almond butter (page 233)

THURSDAY

(1,337 CALORIES)

BREAKFAST (388 CALORIES)
Glass of warm water with fresh lemon juice
Chickpea and coriander crêpes (page 116) with sun-dried tomato and basil hummus (page 227)

SNACK (207 CALORIES)
Green goddess smoothie plus (page 133)

LUNCH (306 CALORIES)
Lime and mint avocado salsa boats (page 231)
Curried cauliflower and sweet potato soup (page 162)

SNACK (108 CALORIES)
Two peanut butter and goji berry protein amazeballs (page 239)

DINNER (290 CALORIES)
Three spicy cauliflower and corn cakes (page 184)
Green salad dressed with balsamic vinegar and lemon juice

TRYPTOPHAN SNACK (38 CALORIES)
250ml warm unsweetened almond milk with a pinch of cinnamon and a few drops of liquid stevia to sweeten (optional)

FRIDAY

(1,300 CALORIES)

BREAKFAST (217 CALORIES)
Glass of warm water with fresh lemon juice
Supergreen smoothie bowl (page 106)

SNACK (158 CALORIES)
125g fresh blueberries or raspberries
2 tablespoons raw pumpkin seeds

LUNCH (388 CALORIES)
Vegetable pad Thai with a spicy almond sauce (page 205)

SNACK (191 CALORIES)
Chocolate peanut butter protein thickshake (page 153)

DINNER (221 CALORIES)
Chilli san carne (page 195)

TRYPTOPHAN SNACK (125 CALORIES)
18 raw unsalted almonds

SATURDAY

BREAKFAST (337 CALORIES)
Glass of warm water with fresh
lemon juice
Rawnola parfait with raspberry and vanilla
coconut whip (page 102)

SNACK (134 CALORIES)
Green goddess juice (page 134)
125g fresh blueberries, strawberries
or raspberries

LUNCH (126 CALORIES)
Curried cauliflower and sweet potato soup
(page 162)

SNACK (274 CALORIES)
Chia summer berry blast (page 149)

DINNER (265 CALORIES)
Smokey falafel burgers in iceberg lettuce
wraps (page 186)
Ginger, chilli and lime broccoli with
toasted sesame seeds (page 170)

**TRYPTOPHAN SNACK (164
CALORIES)**
Sliced apple with 2 teaspoons almond
butter

SUNDAY

(1,299 CALORIES)

BREAKFAST (348 CALORIES)
Glass of warm water with fresh
lemon juice
Two vanilla protein pancakes (page 111)
with 60g fresh blueberries or raspberries

SNACK (205 CALORIES)
Good to glow mango tango smoothie
(page 141)

LUNCH (288 CALORIES)
Butternut squash and sage risotto
(page 208)

SNACK (103 CALORIES)
Chocolate brownie superfood amazeball
(page 236)

DINNER (271 CALORIES)
Vindaloo vegetables with ginger and lime
cauliflower rice (page 198)

TRYPTOPHAN SNACK (84 CALORIES)
12 raw unsalted almonds

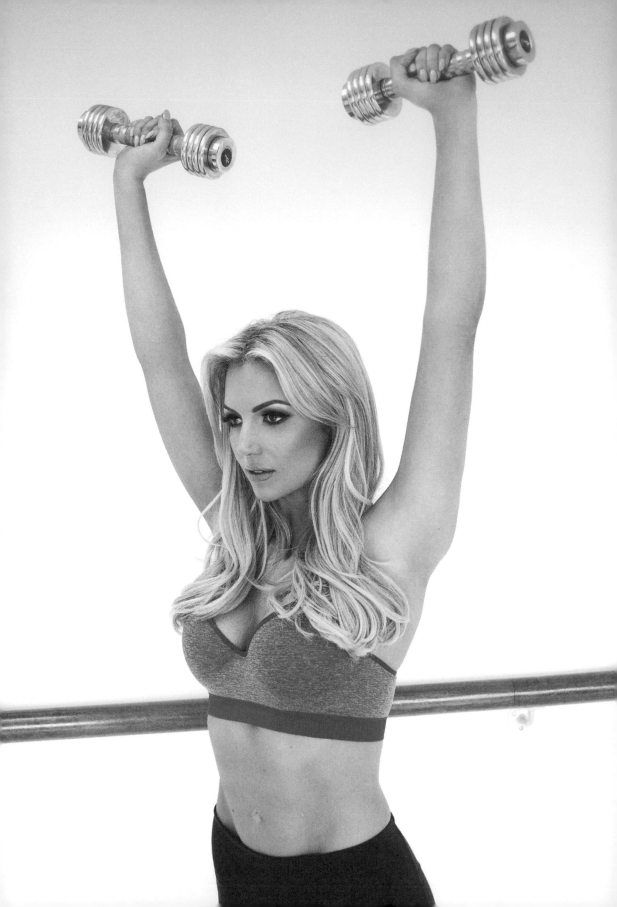

PART 6

FAST FOOD FOR BUSY BODIES

I fully understand how challenging it can be to eat
well when you're busy and under time pressure.
I've designed the majority of the meals, smoothies,
sweet treats and snacks to be simple to make and
affordable, plus most of the ingredients should be
available in one good supermarket.

TAKE 10 INGREDIENTS, MAKE 5 MEALS

My advice is to stock up on a range of dried herbs and spices, coconut oil, coconut milk, oats, quinoa, garlic, nutritional yeast, flours, beans and legumes, nuts, seeds and nut butters to have on hand when you haven't had time to shop for fresh produce.

Bring this list with you the next time you're in the supermarket with limited time and meal inspiration. Once you have the basics, you can play around with using different herbs and spices to flavour your meals.

10 INGREDIENTS

4 large sweet potatoes
2 tins or cartons of cooked chickpeas
2 large heads of cauliflower
1 packet of quinoa
1 packet of split red lentils
1 packet of split yellow peas
1 bag of carrots
1 bag of red onions
1 tube of tomato purée
3 tins of low-fat coconut milk

5 MEALS

Coconut curried quinoa with cheesy roast cauliflower (page 201)
Curried cauliflower and sweet potato soup (page 162)
Carrot, coconut and red lentil soup (page 160)
Smoky falafel burgers (page 186)
Baked sweet potato noodles with red and yellow dahl (page 175)

PART 7

EAT
YOURSELF
FIT RECIPES

 Antioxidant-rich food

 Low-calorie food

 Energy-boosting food

 Muscle-building food

 Good mood food

 Sleep-enhancing food

Please note: The calorie and nutrient content of each recipe are estimates made as closely as possible based on available ingredients.

FUEL YOUR DAY: ENERGY BREAKFASTS

Fitness tip

It's a good idea to include some PROTEIN in your breakfast every day for muscle recovery and repair to help build lean, strong limbs and to stabilise blood sugar levels. This means that you're less likely to experience mid-morning munchies and reach for a sugary or fatty snack to keep you going until lunch.

I love to incorporate AMINO ACIDS into my breakfast by adding nuts, seeds, nut butters and a scoop of high-quality protein powder to smoothies and smoothie bowls.

Peanut Butter and Strawberry Chia Jam Overnight Oats

SERVES 1 | PER SERVING OF OATS: 340 CALORIES | 12G PROTEIN | 36G CARBS | 16.5G FAT
PER JAR OF JAM (USING LIQUID STEVIA TO SWEETEN): 146 CALORIES | 4.3G PROTEIN
20G CARBS | 6.6G FAT

FOR THE OATS:

125ml unsweetened almond milk

1 tbsp whole chia seeds

1 tbsp smooth or crunchy peanut butter (aim to buy organic brands that are free from added sugar and palm oil)

1 tsp vanilla extract or powder

4–5 drops of liquid stevia, to taste (optional)

45g gluten-free porridge oats

FOR THE STRAWBERRY CHIA JAM:

150g fresh strawberries, hulled and sliced in half

2 tbsp whole chia seeds

1 tbsp pure maple syrup or honey or 5–6 drops of liquid stevia (optional)

1 tsp fresh lemon juice

cold water, as required

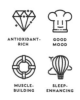

ANTIOXIDANT-RICH   GOOD MOOD   MUSCLE-BUILDING   SLEEP-ENHANCING

I'm a big fan of overnight oats, as they're so simple to make and only require a few key ingredients. They're also ideal for warmer weather as they're served chilled and are perfect for busy people on the go. If you're training before work, make these in a jar the night before and bring them with you for a pre-gym boost or a post-training recovery power breakfast. They contain an ideal combination of complex carbs, protein, omega-3 fats and antioxidants for muscle recovery and repair. They also make a great family breakfast option.

1   First make the chia jam. Place the strawberries, chia seeds, sweetener, if using, and lemon juice in a blender. Blend on a medium to high speed until a jam consistency is achieved, adding 1 tablespoon of cold water at a time to blend as needed.

2   Transfer the mixture to a small saucepan and cook over a medium heat until it begins to bubble. Reduce the heat and allow the jam to simmer gently for 5–6 minutes, until the chia seeds begin to thicken it up.

3   Remove from the heat and pour into a clean glass jar. Allow it to cool before serving. The jam can be stored in the jar with a secure lid in the fridge for up to a week.

4   Place the almond milk, chia seeds, peanut butter, vanilla and stevia, if using, in a glass jar or small bowl and mix together with a spoon. Add the oats and mix well until they're all covered in the almond milk mixture. Top with a generous tablespoon of the strawberry chia jam.

5   If using a jar, screw on the lid securely and leave to chill overnight in the fridge or for at least 6 hours. If using a bowl, cover it with cling film before refrigerating.

6   When you're ready to eat, stir in the strawberry chia jam and enjoy chilled. Overnight oats can be stored in the fridge for up to two days.

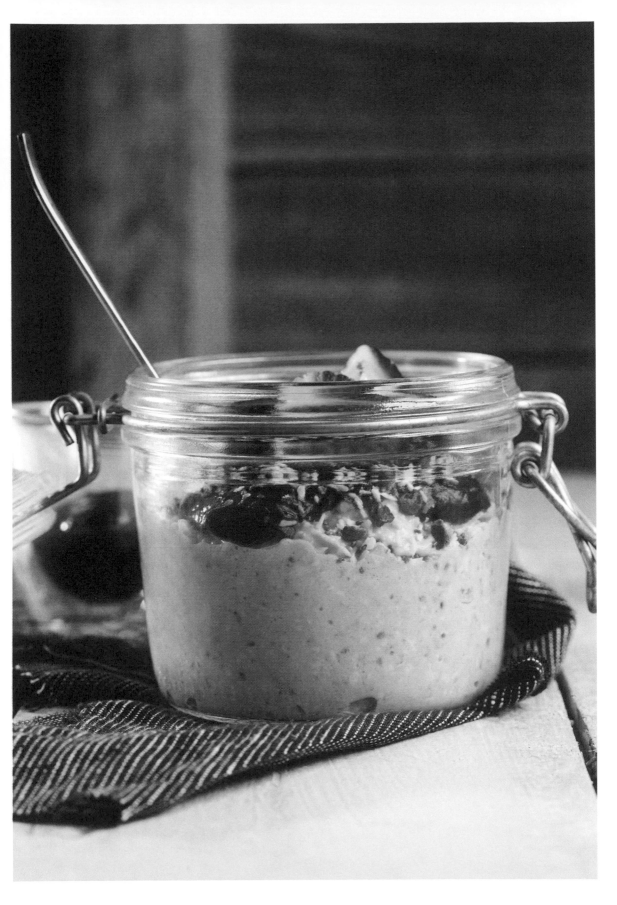

Creamy Millet Power Porridge

SERVES 2 | PER SERVING: 276 CALORIES | 6.8G PROTEIN | 41.6G CARBS | 9.8G FAT

90g millet

500ml cold water

250ml low-fat coconut milk, plus extra to serve

2 tsp vanilla extract or powder

1 tsp ground cinnamon

6–8 drops of liquid stevia (optional)

2 tbsp chopped pecans

125g fresh raspberries or blueberries, to serve

GOOD MOOD   MUSCLE-BUILDING

SLEEP-ENHANCING

Millet isn't just bird food! This creamy, fluffy and mild-tasting grain is actually a seed. It's naturally gluten free and relatively low in calories too. It contains B vitamins to help improve energy levels, particularly vitamin B6 to boost your mood, plus all the essential amino acids to support muscle repair and growth. It's a rich source of magnesium to help relax your nervous system, promote calmness and restful sleep and help to prevent post-workout muscle tightness. As it readily absorbs different flavours, millet works well in main meals and as a porridge. I use pecans as a topping because they contain zinc, vitamin B6 and omega-3 fat, which are important for supporting a happy, positive mindset.

1 Preheat the oven to 190°C.
2 Rinse the millet in a sieve under cold running water. Pour the water and coconut milk into a small saucepan, add the millet and bring it to the boil for 2–3 minutes, stirring regularly.
3 Lower the heat to medium and allow it to simmer for 8–10 minutes, partially covered with a lid, until the liquid has almost boiled off. Remove the lid and stir until the remaining liquid boils off and it has reached a consistency similar to porridge. If it's too dry, stir in a little more coconut milk or water. Add the vanilla and cinnamon to the millet porridge and stir it in along with the liquid stevia, if using.
4 While the millet cooks, spread out the pecans on a small baking tray and toast in the oven for a few minutes, until golden brown. Remove from the oven and set aside.
5 Spoon the millet porridge into two serving bowls. Top with the toasted pecans, fresh berries and an extra dash of coconut milk, if desired.

Energising Apple and Cinnamon Bircher Muesli

SERVES 1 | PER SERVING: 397 CALORIES | 11.6G PROTEIN | 49.8G CARBS | 18.2G FAT

40g gluten-free porridge oats

½ red or green apple, grated

125ml unsweetened almond milk, plus extra for serving

2 tbsp coconut milk yogurt (optional)

1 tbsp unsweetened desiccated coconut

1 tbsp unsweetened dried cranberries

1 tbsp flaxseeds

1 tbsp pumpkin seeds

1 tbsp flaked almonds

1 tsp ground cinnamon

fresh berries or strawberry chia jam (page 98), to serve

ENERGY-BOOSTING   GOOD MOOD

SLEEP-ENHANCING

This easy and nourishing breakfast is one of my favourite ways to start the day. The magical mixture of seeds, nuts, oats and fruit makes it an incredibly energising breakfast. Seeds contain essential omega-3 fatty acids and a wide range of important minerals, including calcium for bone health and muscle function, zinc to support your immune and reproductive systems, iron to maintain good energy levels and magnesium to promote relaxation. This muesli also contains the amino acid tryptophan, vitamin B6 and zinc to support the manufacture of serotonin and a happy, calm mood.

1   Combine all the ingredients in a mixing bowl except for the fresh berries or chia jam and mix well. Taste and add more cinnamon if desired. Cover the bowl and refrigerate overnight to allow the ingredients to soak together.

2   When ready to serve, add a dash of almond milk and top with fresh berries or strawberry chia jam.

Rawnola Parfait with Raspberry and Vanilla Coconut Whip

SERVES 2 | PER SERVING OF RAWNOLA: 337 CALORIES | 11.8G PROTEIN | 33G CARBS | 20.6G FAT
PER SERVING OF RASPBERRY AND VANILLA COCONUT WHIP (2 TBSP): 138 CALORIES
1.9G PROTEIN | 11G CARBS | 10.9G FAT

FOR THE RAWNOLA:

6 tbsp buckwheat groats or gluten-free oats

4 tbsp unsweetened desiccated coconut

2 tbsp whole chia seeds

2 tbsp whole raw almonds

2 tbsp pumpkin seeds

4 tsp almond or hazelnut butter

2 tsp ground cinnamon

½ tsp ground nutmeg

FOR THE RASPBERRY AND VANILLA COCONUT WHIP:

200g coconut milk yogurt or 1 x 400ml tin of full-fat coconut milk, chilled overnight in the fridge

150g fresh raspberries, rinsed (set a few aside to decorate the parfait)

2 tsp vanilla extract or powder

4–5 drops of liquid stevia to sweeten (optional)

This makes the perfect quick and easy breakfast or anytime snack for those following a lower-carb diet. It's packed with healthy fats, fibre and easily assimilated amino acids for muscle recovery and repair, plus those all-important antioxidants found in the cacao nibs and raspberries for protecting your cells from everyday wear and tear.

1 Place all the rawnola ingredients in a food processor fitted with an S blade or a blender and combine until the mixture is crumbly. Set aside.

2 If you're using tinned coconut milk, carefully open it without shaking it. The firm coconut cream should have separated from the coconut water so that you can spoon it out. Place the coconut milk yogurt or cream, raspberries, vanilla and the stevia, if using, in a blender or food processor and blend until smooth and creamy.

3 Layer the parfait ingredients in a glass jar or bowl, starting with the rawnola, then the coconut whip. Repeat until full. Top with a few fresh raspberries and serve. Any leftovers will keep in an airtight container in the fridge for up to two days.

ANTIOXIDANT-RICH   GOOD MOOD

MUSCLE-BUILDING

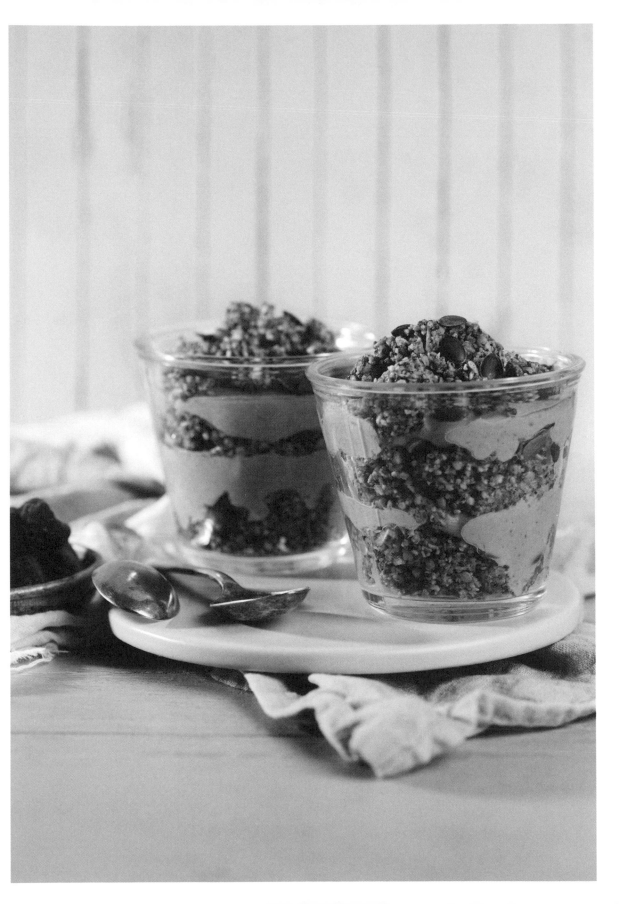

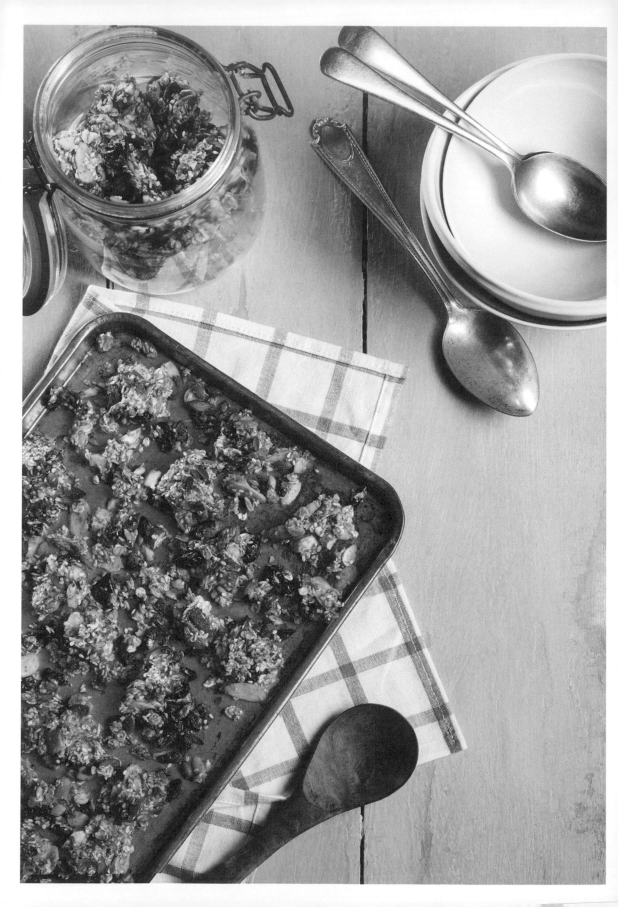

Crunchy Cherry and Coconut Granola Clusters

SERVES 6 | PER SERVING: 348 CALORIES | 11G PROTEIN | 38.6G CARBS | 19.3G FAT

coconut oil, to grease

1 ripe medium banana

1 tbsp pure maple syrup
or honey

1 tbsp tahini

100g gluten-free porridge oats
or quinoa flakes

80g unsweetened dried
cherries (raisins or dried
cranberries make a
good alternative)

65g chopped almonds

55g flaked almonds

4 tbsp unsweetened desiccated
coconut

4 tbsp goji berries

3 tbsp pumpkin seeds

2 tbsp sunflower seeds

2 tbsp milled flaxseeds

2 tbsp sesame seeds

2 tsp ground cinnamon

2 tsp vanilla extract or powder

ENERGY-   GOOD
BOOSTING   MOOD

MUSCLE-
BUILDING

Granola is a tasty and popular breakfast, yet the shop-bought versions tend to be packed with refined sugar, vegetable oil, preservatives and other less-than-healthy ingredients for your skin and waistline. This filling version is full of nourishing and energy-boosting seeds, nuts, unsweetened dried berries, tahini, cinnamon and vanilla for a deliciously nutty, rich taste, and it uses ripe banana in place of oil to reduce the calorie content. I love a handful of this crunchy granola sprinkled on top of smoothies or simply eaten with a splash of ice-cold almond milk.

1 Preheat the oven to 180°C. Line a large baking tray with non-stick baking paper or lightly grease it with coconut oil.

2 Place the banana in a large mixing bowl and mash with a fork, then add the maple syrup and tahini and stir until well mixed. Add all the remaining ingredients and mix until a thick, sticky mixture forms. Add a dash of unsweetened almond milk if the mixture seems too dry.

3 Spread the granola onto the baking tray and toast it in the oven for 15–20 minutes, until golden brown. Stir the granola after 8–10 minutes to ensure it toasts fully and evenly.

4 Remove from the oven and allow the granola to cool for 10 minutes before serving. Store the granola in an airtight container in a cool place for up to three days.

Supergreen Smoothie Bowl

SERVES 1 | PER SERVING: 217 CALORIES | 4.9G PROTEIN | 34.3G CARBS | 9.5G FAT

125ml unsweetened
almond milk

2 handfuls of baby spinach

1 handful of kale, tough
stems removed

80g fresh or frozen
pineapple chunks

juice of ½ lime

¼ ripe avocado

½ ripe banana, fresh or frozen

¼ cucumber

1 tsp wheatgrass powder
(optional)

4–5 drops of liquid stevia to
sweeten (optional)

2–3 ice cubes

TO SERVE:

coconut flakes

fresh berries

fresh figs, quartered

dragon fruit, sliced

chia seeds

cacao nibs

I'm a big advocate of eating leafy green veggies with every meal to avail of their powerful cleansing and energising properties and their huge spectrum of vitamins, minerals and protective phytonutrients. This supergreen smoothie bowl is a great way to enjoy all the goodness of spinach, kale and avocado, sweetened with fruit to hide any 'green' taste.

1 Place all the smoothie bowl ingredients into a blender and blitz until smooth.
2 Pour into a bowl and top with coconut flakes, fresh berries, fresh figs, dragon fruit, chia seeds and cacao nibs. Any leftovers can be stored in an airtight container in the fridge for two or three days.

ANTIOXIDANT-
RICH

ENERGY-
BOOSTING

MUSCLE-
BUILDING

LOW-
CALORIE

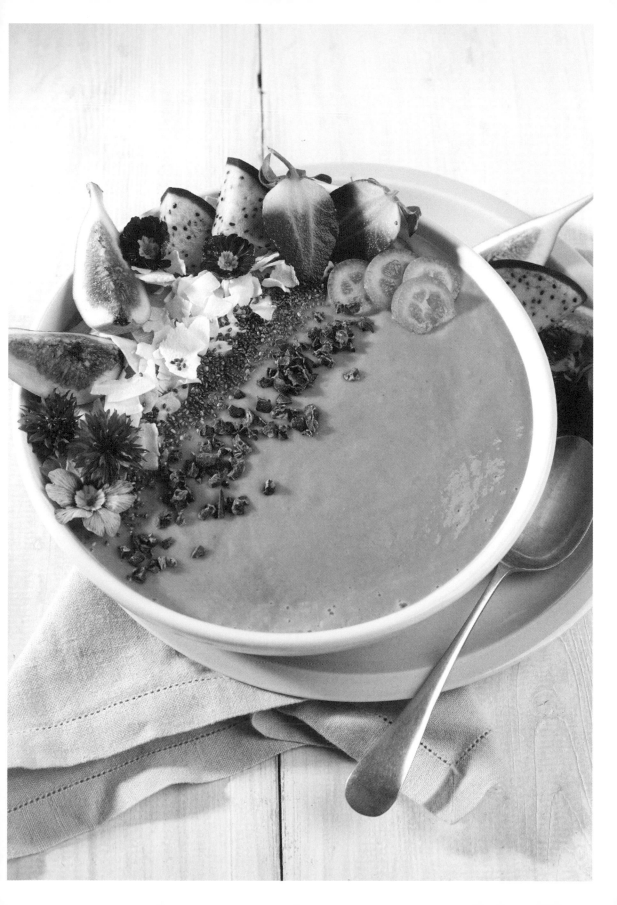

Creamy Cacao Smoothie Bowl with Buckwheat Chocolate Pops

SERVES 1 | PER SERVING OF BUCKWHEAT CHOCOLATE POPS (⅓ OF THE RECIPE): 565 CALORIES
11.6G PROTEIN | 61.6G CARBS | 34.1G FAT
PER SERVING OF SMOOTHIE BOWL: 302 CALORIES | 21.5G PROTEIN |
38.9G CARBS | 9.8G FAT

FOR THE BUCKWHEAT CHOCOLATE POPS:

165g buckwheat groats

80g unsweetened desiccated coconut

3 tbsp raw cacao powder

2 tsp ground cinnamon

2 tbsp coconut oil, melted

2 tbsp pure maple syrup or honey

2 tbsp smooth almond butter

FOR THE CREAMY CACAO SMOOTHIE BOWL:

125ml unsweetened almond milk or low-fat coconut milk

1 frozen banana

1 scoop of Sunwarrior chocolate protein powder (optional)

1 tbsp ground flaxseeds

1 tbsp raw cacao powder

1 tsp raw unsalted almond butter

1 tsp vanilla extract or powder

3–4 drops of liquid stevia, to sweeten (optional)

This is a rich chocolate breakfast using whole ingredients. The buckwheat chocolate pops add a delicious crunch to the smoothie bowl, which is filled with protein, omega-3 fat and antioxidants to keep you feeling full and satisfied all morning. The smoothie bowl serves one but the chocolate pops recipe makes enough for up to three people or it can be enjoyed over a few days.

1   Preheat the oven to 180°C. Line a large baking tray with non-stick baking paper.

2   Combine the buckwheat groats with the coconut, cacao powder and cinnamon in a large mixing bowl.

3   In a separate smaller bowl, mix together the melted coconut oil, maple syrup and almond butter until smooth. Pour the wet ingredients into the bowl with the dry ingredients and mix until it's all well combined.

4   Spread the buckwheat pops on the lined baking tray and bake in the oven for 20–25 minutes, until it's crispy. Allow to cool for 10 minutes before serving.

5   Meanwhile, place all the smoothie bowl ingredients into a blender, beginning with the almond milk. Blend on a high speed until smooth and creamy. Transfer the smoothie to a serving bowl, top with the buckwheat pops and serve.

6   Any leftover buckwheat pops can be stored in an airtight container at room temperature for up to three days. The smoothie can be stored in the fridge for two or three days.

ANTIOXIDANT-RICH   GOOD MOOD

MUSCLE-BUILDING

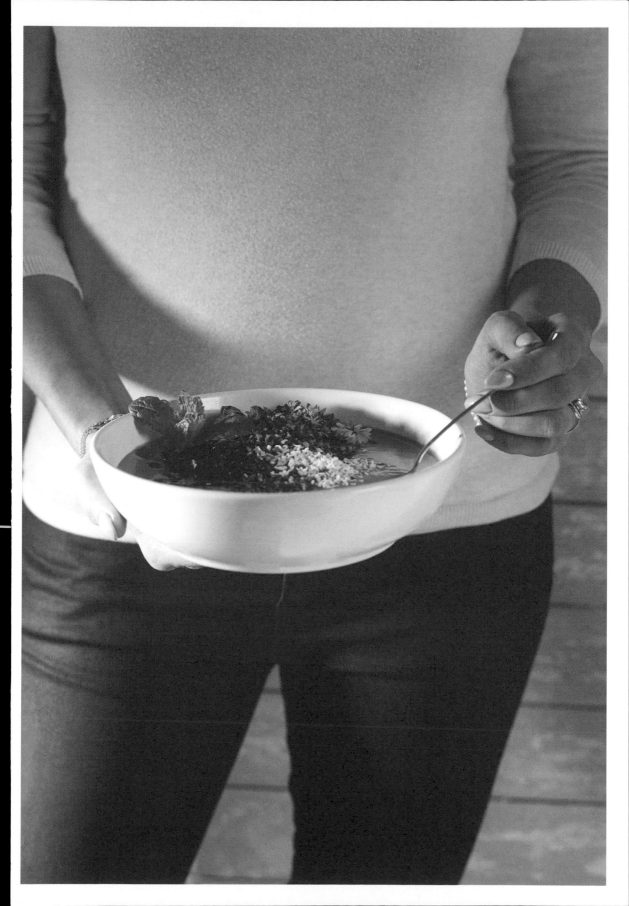

Creamy Chia Pudding with Raspberry Coulis

SERVES 1 | PER SERVING: 270 CALORIES | 7.8G PROTEIN | 28G CARBS | 16.1G FAT

3 heaped tbsp whole
chia seeds

250ml low-fat coconut milk
or unsweetened almond milk

100g fresh raspberries

1 tsp vanilla extract or powder

dash of unsweetened
almond milk

4–5 drops of liquid stevia to
sweeten (optional)

1 tbsp unsweetened
desiccated coconut

ANTIOXIDANT-
RICH   ENERGY-
              BOOSTING

GOOD   MUSCLE-
MOOD   BUILDING

Breakfasts don't get more simple and nourishing than a bowl of chia pudding with an array of tasty toppings. Chia pudding is one of my favourite breakfasts, as it's full of amazing nutrients for your skin, hair and body. It's also a super food for anyone trying to lose a few pounds, because the seeds swell in liquid up to 15 times their own size. This helps to keep you feeling full, well hydrated and far less likely to reach for an unhealthy mid-morning snack. Chia seeds are a good source of omega-3 fat, amino acids, fibre and essential minerals, including iron and calcium.

1   Place the chia seeds in a bowl and pour the coconut or almond milk over them to submerge the seeds. Stir them well and set aside for 10 minutes to soak up all the liquid. You may need to mix them after a few minutes to ensure all the seeds are soaked.

2   Place the raspberries in a small mixing bowl and add the vanilla, a dash of almond milk and the liquid stevia, if using. Use a fork to mash the raspberries, then mix well with the vanilla, almond milk and stevia to make a coulis.

3   Stir the chia pudding once more, ensuring all the liquid has been absorbed by the seeds. Top with the raspberry coulis and a sprinkle of desiccated coconut. Any leftovers can be stored in an airtight container in the fridge for up to three days.

Vanilla Protein Pancakes

MAKES 6 PANCAKES | PER PLAIN PANCAKE: 157 CALORIES | 7.5G PROTEIN | 20G CARBS | 2.8G FAT

180g gluten-free self-raising flour (I use Doves Farm brand)

2 scoops of Sunwarrior vanilla protein powder

625ml unsweetened almond milk

2 tbsp milled chia seeds

2 tsp vanilla extract or powder

coconut oil, to cook

fresh berries, to serve

1 tbsp pure maple syrup or honey, to serve (optional)

ENERGY-BOOSTING   LOW-CALORIE

MUSCLE-BUILDING

I love these light, fluffy, vanilla-flavoured pancakes with fresh berries. They make a satisfying post-workout meal filled with fibre, amino acids and omega-3 fats, nourishing every cell in your body to help keep you healthy and strong.

1   Place the flour, protein powder, almond milk, milled chia seeds and vanilla in a blender and combine until a thick batter forms.

2   Heat a little coconut oil in a frying pan set over a medium heat. When it begins to bubble, place a tablespoon of batter into the middle of the pan. I like to smooth it out to form a neat circle. Cook until the edges begin to rise, then flip it over and cook until both sides are golden brown. They cook very quickly.

3   Top with fresh berries and maple syrup, if using, and serve hot. Any leftovers can be stored in an airtight container in the fridge for up to three days.

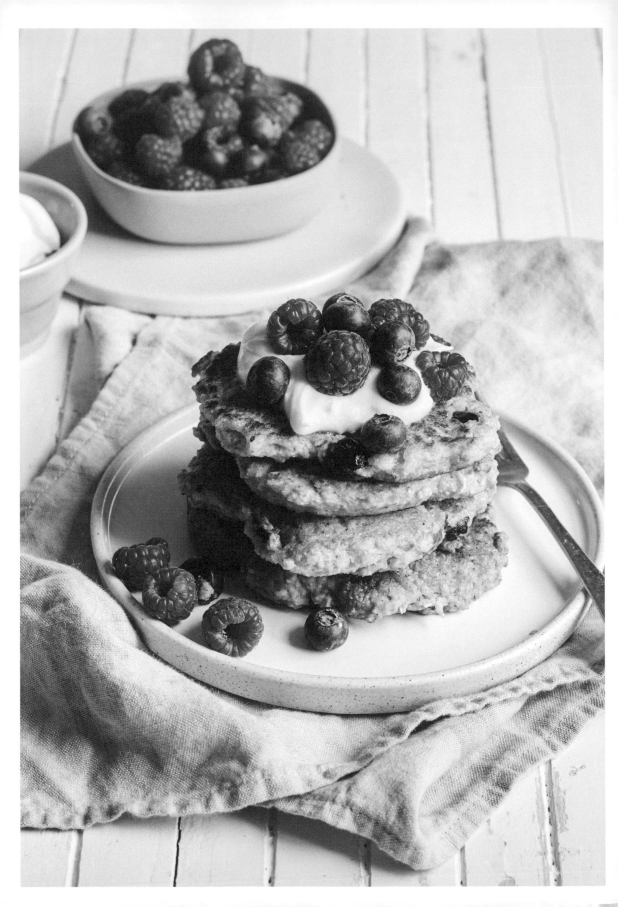

Very Berry Oatmeal Pancakes with Vanilla Coconut Cream

MAKES 6 PANCAKES | PER SERVING (2 PANCAKES): 262 CALORIES
8.3G PROTEIN | 43G CARBS | 5.9G FAT
PER SERVING OF VANILLA COCONUT CREAM (2 TBSP): 99 CALORIES
1G PROTEIN | 2G CARBS | 10.4G FAT

1 tbsp ground flaxseeds

3 tbsp cold water

155g gluten-free oats

1 ripe banana

250ml unsweetened almond milk

1 tsp vanilla extract

½ tsp gluten-free baking powder

2 tbsp fresh blueberries, plus extra to serve

2 tbsp fresh raspberries, plus extra to serve

coconut oil, to cook

FOR THE COCONUT CREAM:

1 x 400ml tin of full-fat coconut milk, chilled overnight in the fridge

1 tsp vanilla extract or powder

ENERGY-BOOSTING   GOOD MOOD

These tasty oat-based pancakes contain sweet pops of antioxidant-rich berries and make the perfect dish for a lazy Sunday morning brunch or a post-workout energy booster. Oats are a good source of slow-release energy and fibre, while the ground flaxseeds increase the fibre content of these pancakes even more. Oats also contain iron to boost energy levels and magnesium to support nervous system health.

1   First make the flax 'egg' by placing the ground flaxseeds in a small bowl and adding the cold water. Mix well and leave to set for 5 minutes.

2   Place the oats, banana, almond milk, vanilla extract, baking powder and flax 'egg' in a blender and combine until a thick batter forms. Transfer the batter to a bowl and stir in the blueberries and raspberries.

3   Heat some coconut oil in a frying pan set over a medium heat. Spoon 2 tablespoons of the batter into the centre of the pan to make each pancake. Allow them to cook for about 60 seconds, then gently lift up the edges with a spatula and flip over to cook on the other side for another 60 seconds, until golden brown.

4   Once all the pancakes have been cooked, allow them to cool for a few minutes while you prepare the coconut cream. Carefully open the tin of chilled coconut milk without shaking it, as the thick cream should have separated from the coconut water. Spoon out the coconut cream into a bowl. Add the vanilla and use a hand-held whisk to whisk the coconut cream until light and fluffy.

5   Serve the warm pancakes with a dollop of the coconut cream on top and scatter over the fresh berries. Any leftovers can be stored in an airtight container in the fridge for two or three days.

Spiced Apple and Cranberry Pancakes

MAKES 8 PANCAKES | PER PANCAKE (WITHOUT SYRUP): 97 CALORIES | 2.1G PROTEIN
19.5G CARBS | 1.5G FAT

125g gluten-free self-raising flour (I use Doves Farm brand)

375ml unsweetened almond milk

2 heaped tbsp milled chia seeds

2 tsp ground cinnamon

½ tsp ground nutmeg

coconut oil, to cook

TO SERVE:

1 large or 2 small apples, cored and grated

4 tbsp unsweetened dried cranberries

1 tsp ground cinnamon

drizzle of pure maple syrup or honey (optional)

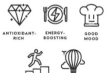

ANTIOXIDANT-RICH   ENERGY-BOOSTING   GOOD MOOD

LOW-CALORIE   SLEEP-ENHANCING

These fluffy, lightly spiced pancakes are based on gluten-free flour and fibre-rich chia seeds. The naturally sweet grated apple and cranberries deliver a blast of immune-boosting vitamin C and antioxidants.

1   Place the flour, almond milk, milled chia seeds, cinnamon and nutmeg in a blender and blend on a high speed until a smooth batter forms.

2   Heat a little coconut oil in a frying pan set over a medium-high heat. When it begins to bubble, pour in enough batter to make a thin, medium-sized pancake. When the edges of the pancake start to detach from the base of the pan, use a spatula to lift the pancake free from the pan and carefully flip it over. Cook it on the other side until golden brown.

3   Place on a plate topped with a piece of kitchen paper to mop up any extra oil. Continue cooking until all the batter is gone, then top with grated apple, dried cranberries, a sprinkle of ground cinnamon and a drizzle of maple syrup if you like. Any leftovers can be stored in an airtight container in the fridge for two or three days.

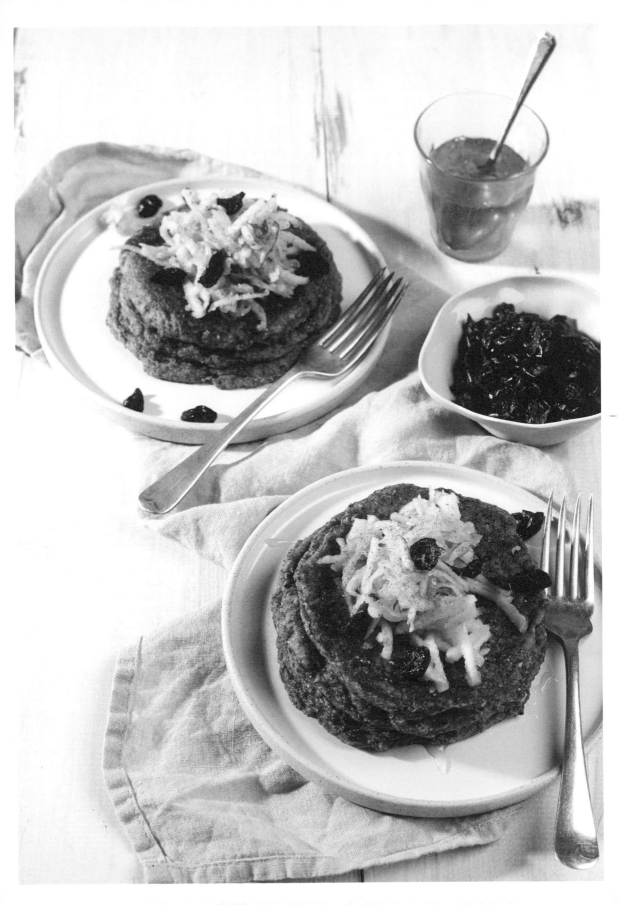

Chickpea and Coriander Crêpes

MAKES 4–5 | PER SERVING (2 CRÊPES): 190 CALORIES | 10.3G PROTEIN | 25.6G CARBS | 5.1G FAT

90g chickpea flour (also called gram flour)

375ml water

2 tbsp ground flaxseeds

1 tsp smoked paprika

1 tsp ground cumin

1 handful of fresh coriander leaves, chopped, or 1 tsp ground coriander

pinch of dried chilli flakes (optional)

sea salt and freshly ground black pepper

coconut oil, to cook

TO SERVE:

hummus

avocado or guacamole

fresh rocket leaves

cherry tomatoes

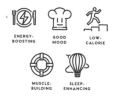

ENERGY-BOOSTING   GOOD MOOD   LOW-CALORIE

MUSCLE-BUILDING   SLEEP-ENHANCING

These crêpes are ideal if you enjoy a savoury breakfast. They're so simple to make and they cook even quicker than regular pancakes. Made with chickpea flour, they're light yet high in protein and fibre, iron, folate, zinc and magnesium amongst many other vital nutrients. They taste delicious served with hummus, avocado and fresh rocket leaves.

1   Place the chickpea flour, water, flaxseeds, spices and seasoning in a blender and blend until a smooth batter forms. Add a little extra water if it's too thick. The thicker the batter is, the thicker the crêpes will be.

2   Melt ½ teaspoon of coconut oil in a frying pan set over a medium heat, then gently pour in the batter to the size of pancake you prefer. Allow it to cook for about 60 seconds before flipping it over with a spatula and cooking for another 60 seconds on the other side. These crêpes cook faster than regular pancakes. Repeat until the batter has been used up.

3   Serve warm with hummus, avocado, rocket and cherry tomatoes. Any leftovers can be stored in an airtight container in the fridge for three or four days.

Seeded Cranberry Muesli Bars

MAKES 10–12 BARS | PER BAR: 118 CALORIES | 3.5G PROTEIN | 11.6G CARBS | 5.4G FAT

60g gluten-free porridge oats

110g pitted dates, soaked in hot water for 20 minutes to soften

125ml water

80g whole chia seeds

35g raw sunflower seeds

35g raw pumpkin seeds

30g unsweetened dried cranberries, chopped

1 tsp ground cinnamon

1 tsp vanilla extract or powder

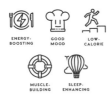

ENERGY-BOOSTING   GOOD MOOD   LOW-CALORIE

MUSCLE-BUILDING   SLEEP-ENHANCING

Muesli in a bar for busy people on the move! These simple bars are filled with oats, seeds and dried cranberries for a nourishing grab-and-go breakfast option or anytime snack. If I'm out and about all day, I carry a wrapped bar around in my bag for hunger emergencies.

1   Preheat the oven to 190°C. Line a medium baking tray with non-stick baking paper.
2   Place the oats in a blender and blend on a high speed for 1–2 minutes, until a fine flour forms. Transfer the oat flour to a large mixing bowl.
3   Add the soaked and drained dates and the water to the blender and blend again until a smooth paste forms. Pour the date paste into the bowl with the oat flour and add all the remaining ingredients. Mix well to combine.
4   Transfer the mixture to the lined baking tray and spread it out, ensuring the surface is as smooth and even as possible. Bake in the oven for 20–25 minutes, until golden brown and firm to touch. Allow the mixture to cool in the baking tray for a few minutes before transferring it to a wire cooling rack for another 10 minutes, then slice into bars. Any leftovers can be stored in an airtight container for three or four days or frozen for up to three months.

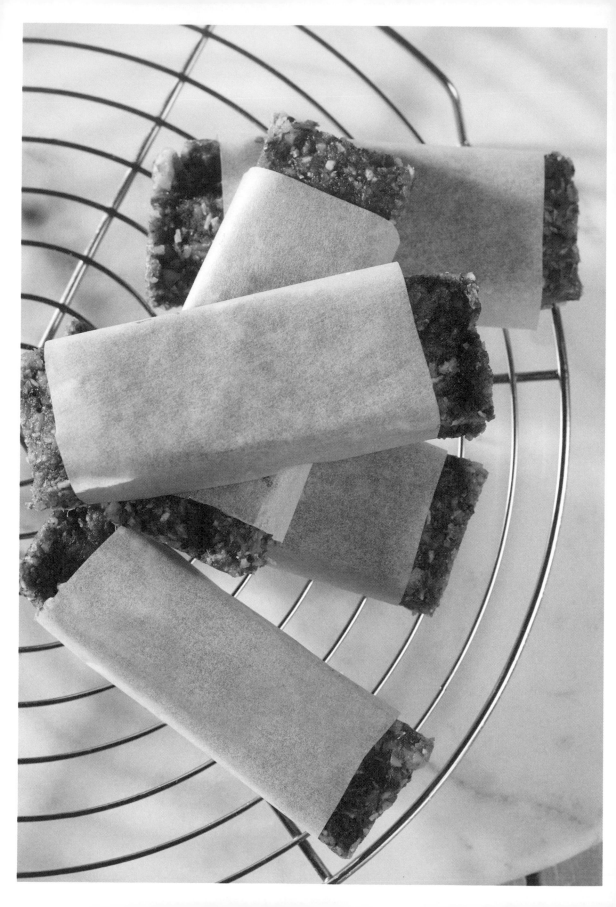

Omega-3 Gingerbread Energy Bars

MAKES 6–8 BARS | PER BAR: 88 CALORIES | 4G PROTEIN | 7G CARBS | 6.6G FAT

150g raw walnut halves

8–10 dried apricots (organic and sulphur free, if possible)

10–12 dates, pitted and soaked in hot water for 20 minutes to soften

2 tbsp unsweetened desiccated or flaked coconut

1 tbsp finely chopped fresh ginger

1 tbsp almond butter

1 tsp ground cinnamon

1 tsp vanilla extract

½ tsp ground nutmeg

ANTIOXIDANT-RICH   ENERGY-BOOSTING

GOOD MOOD   LOW-CALORIE

Omega-3 fatty acids are absolutely essential to include in your everyday diet for their powerful anti-inflammatory properties. They help to keep your skin smooth and are important for maintaining good brain health and regulating hormones. Raw walnuts are one of the best plant-based sources of the nutrient and provide a protein- and fibre-rich base for these energy bars. Fresh ginger helps to support your immune system, improves blood flow and supports healthy digestion. These bars are simple to make and are a tasty quick breakfast or snack on the go.

1   Place the walnuts and apricots in a blender or a food processor fitted with an S blade. Combine until the mixture becomes a coarse flour. Add the soaked and drained dates, coconut, ginger, almond butter, cinnamon, vanilla and nutmeg and blend until the mixture becomes a sticky dough.

2   Press the mixture into a tray lined with non-stick baking paper and chill in the fridge for 30–40 minutes before slicing into squares and serving. Store in an airtight container in the fridge for three or four days.

Almond Butter Chocolate Chip Protein Bars

MAKES 12 BARS | PER BAR: 143 CALORIES | 6.1G PROTEIN | 14.9G CARBS | 7G FAT

200g gluten-free porridge oats

125g smooth or crunchy almond butter

30g (1½ scoops) Sunwarrior vanilla protein powder

10 dates, pitted and soaked in hot water for 20 minutes to soften

2 tsp vanilla extract or powder

7–8 tbsp cold water, to blend

3 tbsp cacao nibs or unsweetened dark chocolate chips

ENERGY-BOOSTING   GOOD MOOD

LOW-CALORIE   MUSCLE-BUILDING

It's important to eat protein with each meal for a healthy metabolism. These bars are an ideal breakfast on the go as they're packed with protein, fibre, healthy fats, complex carbs, an array of vitamins and minerals and the natural energy-boosting goodness of dates. They're also perfect for a post-weightlifting snack to replenish used-up carbohydrate stores and get to work on healing and rebuilding torn muscle fibres.

1   Place the oats in a blender or food processor and blend for 1–2 minutes, until a coarse flour forms. Add the almond butter, protein powder, soaked and drained dates and vanilla and blend for another 30–45 seconds. Slowly add the water while pulsing to combine the mixture into a thick, sticky dough. Transfer to a mixing bowl and stir in the chocolate chips until well distributed.

2   Line a square 20cm x 20cm baking tray with non-stick baking paper and scrape the mixture into it, pressing it down firmly with the back of a spoon to form a smooth, firm layer. Place in the freezer for 20–30 minutes, until firm, then slice into bars. Keep the bars refrigerated in an airtight container for up to five days.

Strawberry and Banana Porridge Bread

MAKES 1 LOAF | PER SLICE (UNSWEETENED): 240 CALORIES | 6.3G PROTEIN | 31G CARBS | 9.9G FAT

4 tbsp ground flaxseeds

8 tbsp cold water

3 ripe bananas

8 medium strawberries

4 tbsp coconut palm sugar,
pure maple syrup or honey
(optional)

2 tsp vanilla extract

4 tbsp coconut oil, melted,
plus extra for greasing

2 level tsp gluten-free
baking powder

400g gluten-free porridge oats

ANTIOXIDANT-RICH   ENERGY-BOOSTING

GOOD MOOD   SLEEP-ENHANCING

This loaf is filled with sweet, juicy fruit, making it a delicious breakfast option and a handy way to use up ripe bananas. Ground flaxseeds and porridge oats blended into a flour form the base of this fibre-rich bread, which helps to boost digestive health. An optimally functioning digestive system benefits you in numerous ways and even helps to prevent a bloated stomach. Oats and bananas both encourage the production of serotonin for a happy mood, and melatonin for peaceful sleep.

1   Preheat the oven to 190°C. Lightly grease a loaf tin with coconut oil or line it with non-stick baking paper.

2   Prepare the flax 'eggs' by mixing the ground flaxseeds with the cold water in a bowl. Set aside.

3   Mash together two of the bananas and all the strawberries in a large mixing bowl until quite smooth but some texture still remains. Add the coconut sugar, if using, and the vanilla and mix well, then stir in the flax 'eggs', melted coconut oil and baking powder and stir until combined.

4   Blend the oats in a food processor or blender until a flour is formed, then fold the flour into the mixture to form a batter. Spoon the batter into the loaf tin and use a spatula to smooth the top. Cut the remaining banana in half and place it across the top to decorate.

5   Bake in the oven for 45–50 minutes, until the top turns golden brown and a knife comes out clean when inserted into the centre. Cool on a wire rack for 10 minutes before serving. The bread can be stored in an airtight container in the fridge for three or four days.

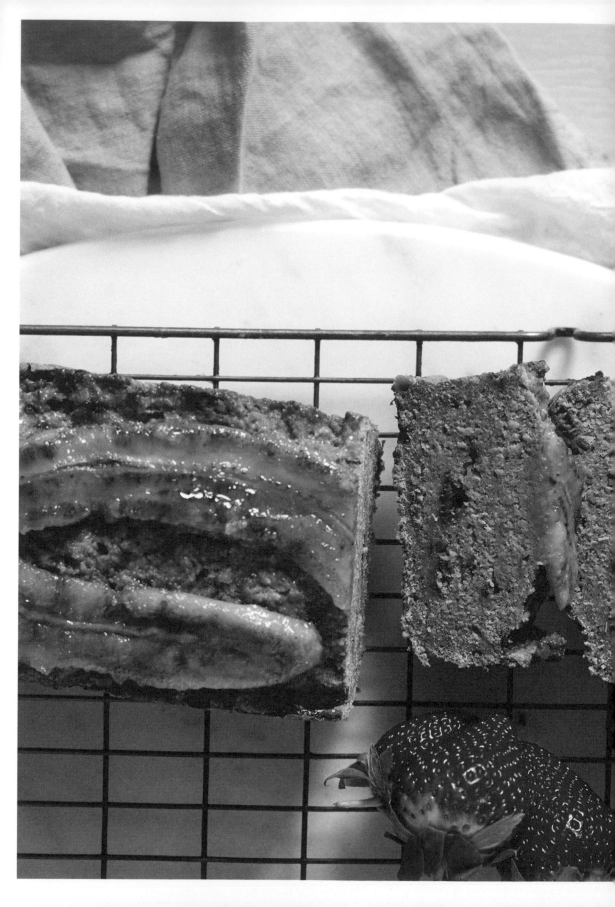

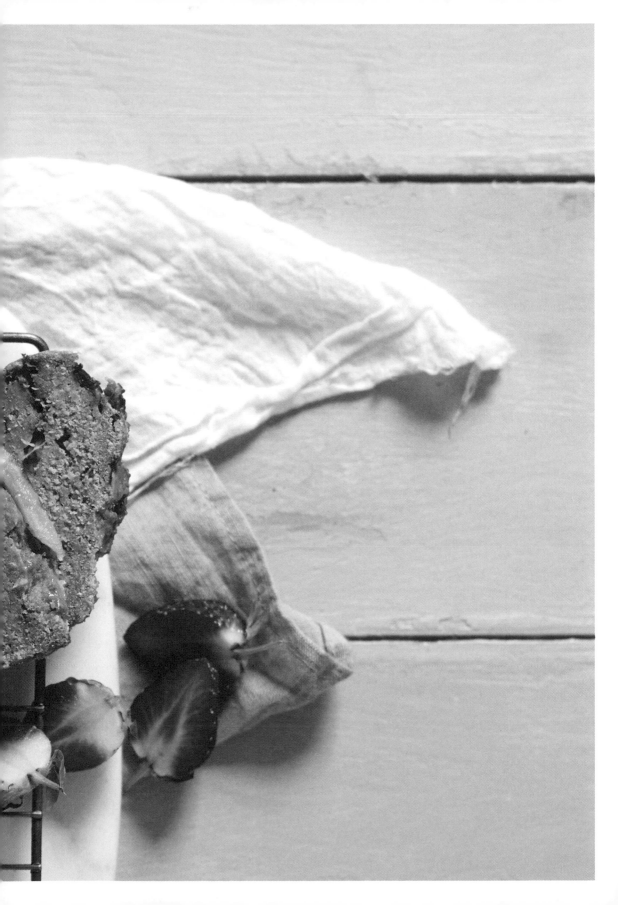

Spiced Sweet Potato Bread

MAKES 1 LOAF | PER SLICE: 155 CALORIES | 4.5G PROTEIN | 22.2G CARBS | 6.4G FAT

coconut oil, to grease

2 medium sweet potatoes, peeled and roughly chopped

2 ripe bananas

250ml unsweetened almond milk

255g gluten-free flour

210g almonds, chopped, plus extra whole almonds to decorate (omit for a nut-free recipe)

100g coconut sugar

4 heaped tbsp coconut flour

3 tbsp milled chia seeds

4 tsp ground cinnamon

4 tsp vanilla extract

2 tsp ground allspice

1¼ tsp gluten-free baking powder

pinch of pink rock salt

ENERGY-
BOOSTING

GOOD
MOOD

LOW-
CALORIE

Sweet potato is an incredibly versatile and nutritious source of filling fibre and complex carbs. It's packed with skin-brightening beta-carotene and it makes a superb alternative to fats and oils in baking. This helps to lower the fat and calorie content of recipes while introducing a soft texture and naturally sweet taste. For this bread I use crunchy almonds to boost its protein and fibre content and plenty of cinnamon for its fragrant flavour and blood sugar control benefits. This bread tastes great spread with nut or seed butter.

1   Preheat the oven to 190°C. Lightly grease a loaf tin with coconut oil.

2   Steam the sweet potatoes for about 10 minutes, until soft. Place the steamed sweet potatoes, bananas and almond milk in a blender and blend until a smooth purée forms. Pour the sweet potato and banana purée into a large mixing bowl and add all the other ingredients. Stir everything together until a thick batter forms.

3   Transfer the batter to the tin, ensuring the top is smooth and even. Decorate with a sprinkle of cinnamon and the whole almonds. Bake in the oven for 25 minutes, until the loaf is golden brown and firm to touch. Allow it to cool for 10 minutes before slicing. Any leftovers should keep in an airtight container in the fridge for up to three days and it can be frozen for up to three months.

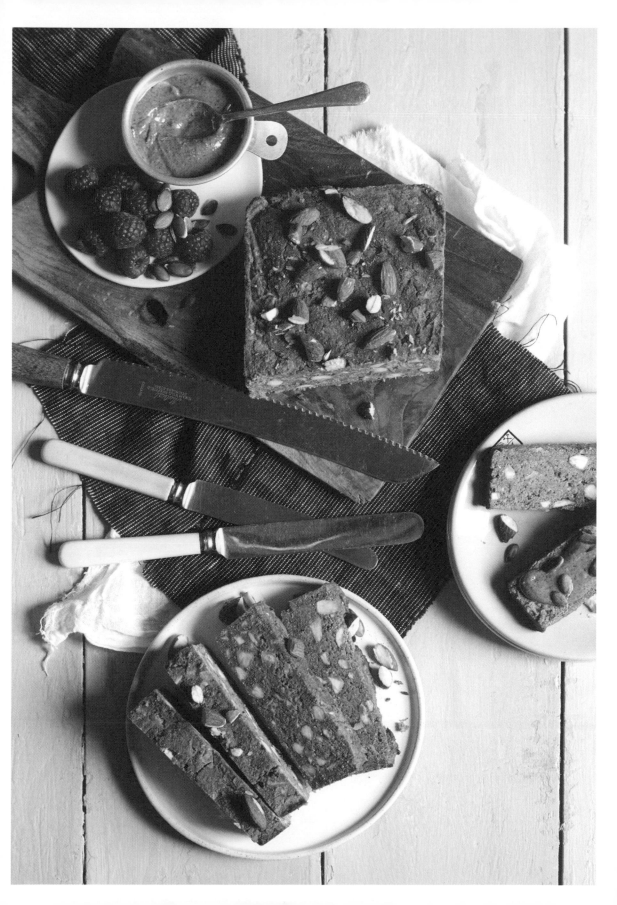

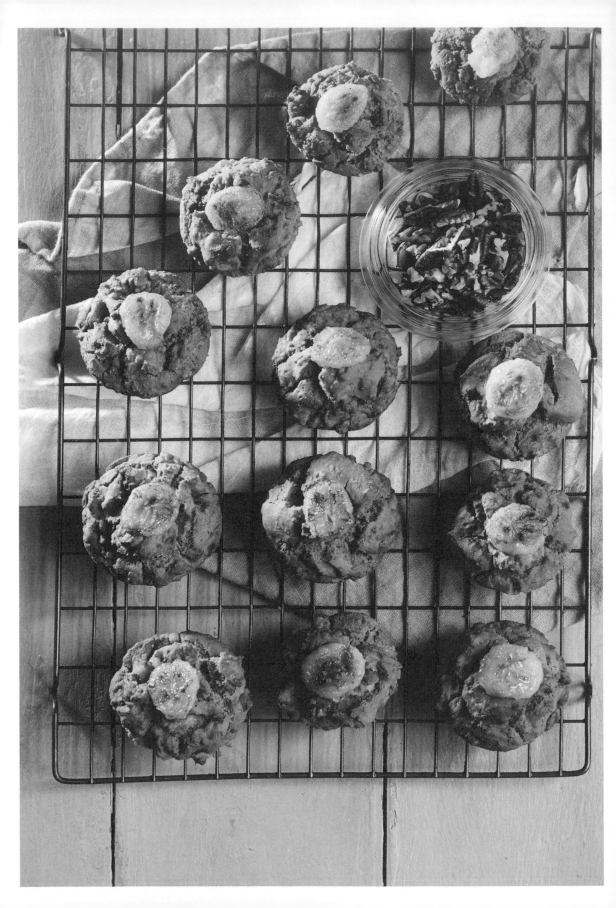

Banana Nut Muffins

MAKES 10–12 MUFFINS | PER MUFFIN: 320 CALORIES | 3.6G PROTEIN | 49.7G CARBS | 13G FAT

250ml unsweetened almond milk

1 tsp raw apple cider vinegar

255g gluten-free all-purpose flour

2½ tsp gluten-free baking powder

¼ tsp gluten-free baking soda

75g coconut sugar

65g coconut oil, melted, plus extra to grease

1 tsp vanilla extract

2 ripe bananas, chopped into small pieces, plus 10–12 slices to decorate

4 tbsp chopped pecans

ENERGY-
BOOSTING

GOOD
MOOD

SLEEP-
ENHANCING

These muffins are the ultimate good mood food. Packed with vitamin B6 and the amino acid tryptophan, bananas help your body to make serotonin, the mood-boosting happy hormone. Sufficient levels of this important neurotransmitter in your brain help to lower cravings for fatty and sugary foods, improve your sleep, increase feelings of contentment and self-confidence and reduce feelings of stress and anxiety. I included the pecans in these muffins because they provide the mineral zinc, an important co-factor in the production of serotonin.

1   Preheat the oven to 190°C. Lightly grease a muffin tray with coconut oil or line with muffin cases.

2   Place the almond milk in a small bowl or glass and stir in the apple cider vinegar. Set aside.

3   Sift the flour, baking powder and baking soda into a large mixing bowl and add the coconut sugar. Combine well.

4   Mix the melted coconut oil with the vanilla extract in a separate bowl, then add the almond milk and vinegar mixture (the milk should have curdled slightly).

5   Add the wet mixture to the dry ingredients in the large bowl and stir together until a thick batter forms. Gently fold in the banana pieces and the chopped nuts and ensure they're evenly distributed.

6   Divide the batter between the muffin cases, then top each muffin with a thin slice of banana and bake for 20–25 minutes, until the muffins turn golden brown and the banana on top starts to caramelise. Allow to cool on a wire cooling rack for 10 minutes before serving. Store in an airtight container in a cool place for two or three days.

Lemon and Blueberry Scones

MAKES 6–8 SCONES | PER SCONE: 251 CALORIES | 2.6G PROTEIN | 32.6G CARBS | 12.8G FAT

1 tbsp ground flaxseeds

3 tbsp cold water

180ml unsweetened almond milk

260g white or brown rice flour or gluten-free plain flour (note: buckwheat flour is not ideal for this recipe)

50g coconut sugar

¾ tbsp gluten-free baking powder

pinch of sea salt

90g coconut oil, at room temperature, plus extra for greasing

60g fresh or frozen blueberries

zest of 1 lemon

ANTIOXIDANT-RICH   ENERGY-BOOSTING

These light and fluffy scones packed with sweet pops of flavour from the lemon zest and antioxidant-rich blueberries are the perfect breakfast or snack on the go and a good option for anybody tempted by sugary pastries in the morning. I have used coconut sugar to gently sweeten them, which is a better alternative to refined sugar, as it's richer in minerals and doesn't cause a spike in your blood sugar levels.

1   Preheat the oven to 190°C. Line a medium baking tray with non-stick baking paper or lightly grease with coconut oil.

2   Prepare the flax 'egg' first by placing the ground flaxseeds into a small bowl and adding the water. Mix well and set aside for 5 minutes. Add the almond milk to the flax 'egg' and use a fork to whisk it in to break up any large lumps of flaxseeds.

3   In a large mixing bowl, combine the flour with the coconut sugar, baking powder and sea salt. Add the coconut oil, using your fingertips to gently break it up into small pieces and distribute it throughout the dry ingredients. Add the flax 'egg' and almond milk combination, mixing until well combined, then gently fold in the blueberries and lemon zest until they're evenly distributed.

4   Lightly flour a clean work surface and use your hands to divide the dough into circular shapes about 2.5cm thick. Place each scone on the lined baking tray and bake in the oven for 20–25 minutes, until golden brown. Allow the scones to cool on a wire rack for 10 minutes before serving. Store any leftovers in an airtight container for up to three days.

Roast Portobello Mushrooms Stuffed with Chilli-Lime Guacamole

SERVES 2 | PER SERVING: 209 CALORIES | 7.4G PROTEIN | 15.9G CARBS | 15.7G FAT

coconut oil, to grease

6 Portobello mushrooms

1 tsp smoked paprika, plus extra to serve

sea salt and freshly ground black pepper

1 small ripe avocado

juice of ½ lime

pinch of dried chilli flakes

ANTIOXIDANT-RICH   GOOD MOOD

LOW-CALORIE

An ideal option for anybody following a low-carb diet, this combination of warm grilled Portobello mushrooms and chilli-lime guacamole is delicious and simple to prepare. Avocados are one of nature's most superior sources of healthy fat, amino acids, antioxidant vitamins A, C and E and essential minerals, including iron to boost energy and potassium for healthy, normal blood pressure. While some dietary fat is essential, avocados are rich in calories. I recommend eating no more than half an avocado a day, unless you're especially active.

1   Preheat the oven to 190°C. Lightly grease a baking tray with coconut oil or line with a sheet of non-stick baking paper.

2   Gently rinse the mushrooms and remove their stalks. Place them on the tray and sprinkle with the smoked paprika, salt and pepper. Roast in the oven for 15–20 minutes, until they begin to shrink slightly and release their juices.

3   While the mushrooms are roasting, slice the avocado in half, remove the stone and use a spoon to scoop the flesh into a bowl. Squeeze in the fresh lime juice and add the chilli flakes, salt and pepper. Use a fork to mash the avocado until smooth.

4   Remove the mushrooms from the oven and allow them to cool for a few minutes before spooning some of the mashed avocado into the centre of each one. Sprinkle with a little extra smoked paprika and serve warm or cold. Any leftovers can be stored in an airtight container in the fridge for up to two days, but the avocado can begin to oxidise and turn brown when exposed to the air, so this is really best eaten on the day it's made.

LIQUID VITALITY

Fitness tip

Blended foods and juices hit your BLOODSTREAM more quickly than solid foods, which means their nutrients get delivered to all your BODY CELLS much faster. That's just one of the reasons why a nutritious, PROTEIN-RICH smoothie makes such a perfect post-workout snack. I always aim to drink a smoothie with some PROTEIN, GREENS and BERRIES after a tough resistance workout to boost my energy and fill my system with all the goodness it needs for repairing and rebuilding my muscles.

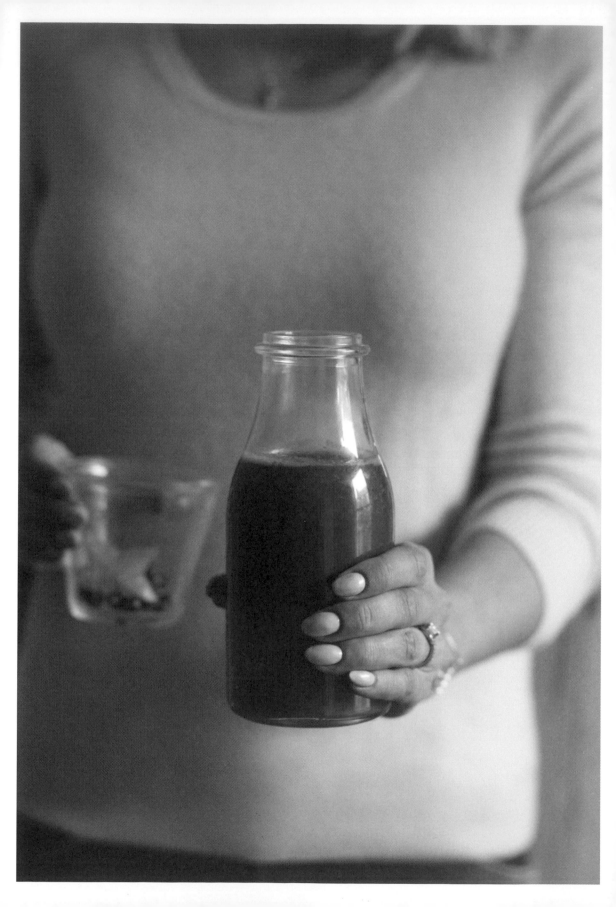

Green Goddess Smoothie Plus

SERVES 2 | PER SERVING: 207 CALORIES | 6.3G PROTEIN | 41G CARBS | 4.3G FAT

125ml cold water

165g pineapple chunks

120g baby spinach, washed well

1 ripe banana, peeled

½ cucumber, chopped into chunks (leave the skin on and buy organic cucumbers if possible)

1 handful of fresh blueberries (use less for a brighter green drink and more for a darker drink)

2 tbsp freshly squeezed lemon or lime juice

2 tbsp hulled hemp seeds, chia seeds or flaxseeds

1 tbsp fresh mint leaves

1 tsp freshly grated ginger

4 ice cubes

4–5 drops of liquid stevia (optional)

ANTIOXIDANT-RICH   ENERGY-BOOSTING

LOW-CALORIE

This is my signature drink and an important part of both the *Eat Yourself Beautiful* and *Eat Yourself Fit* programmes. Even if you don't make any other significant changes to your diet and lifestyle, simply drinking a large glass of this smoothie in the morning at least four times a week will make a noticeable difference to your health, energy levels, digestion, waistline, fitness and immune system. I have incorporated some of the very best foods for younger-looking skin, fat burning and anti-ageing into one drink. It's easy to make in big batches two or three times a week, as it keeps fresh for a few days in the fridge. In this version, I've added seeds for a protein boost, making it an ideal pre- or post-workout smoothie.

1   Add the water to the blender first, followed by the remaining ingredients. Blend until smooth and creamy. Taste and add a few drops of liquid stevia if desired.

2   Serve chilled in a tall glass. You can store any leftovers in the freezer or it keeps fresh in the fridge for two or three days.

Green Goddess Juice

2 cucumbers, cut into medium-sized pieces (leave the skin on and buy organic cucumbers if possible)

60g kale leaves, tough stems removed

60g baby spinach

1 handful of fresh mint leaves

2 tsp freshly grated ginger

1 lime, peeled and halved

ice cubes, for serving

ANTIOXIDANT-RICH   ENERGY-BOOSTING

LOW-CALORIE

This is a highly energising and refreshing minty green juice with ginger and lime. I love green juices because their vast array of vitamins, minerals and phytonutrients are quickly absorbed into your bloodstream, where they deliver their nutrients to every cell in your body for deep cleansing, detoxing and nourishment. I'm not a big fan of juicing fruit because the fibre has been removed and it hits your bloodstream too quickly. This can cause an energy crash, which may affect your mood. If you would like a sweeter green drink, try adding a little puréed banana or blueberries to the juice.

1   Prepare the ingredients and process them through the juicer in the order listed.
2   Serve chilled in a tall glass or jar with a couple of ice cubes. It's best to drink this juice as soon as possible after pressing, but it can be frozen for up to three months.

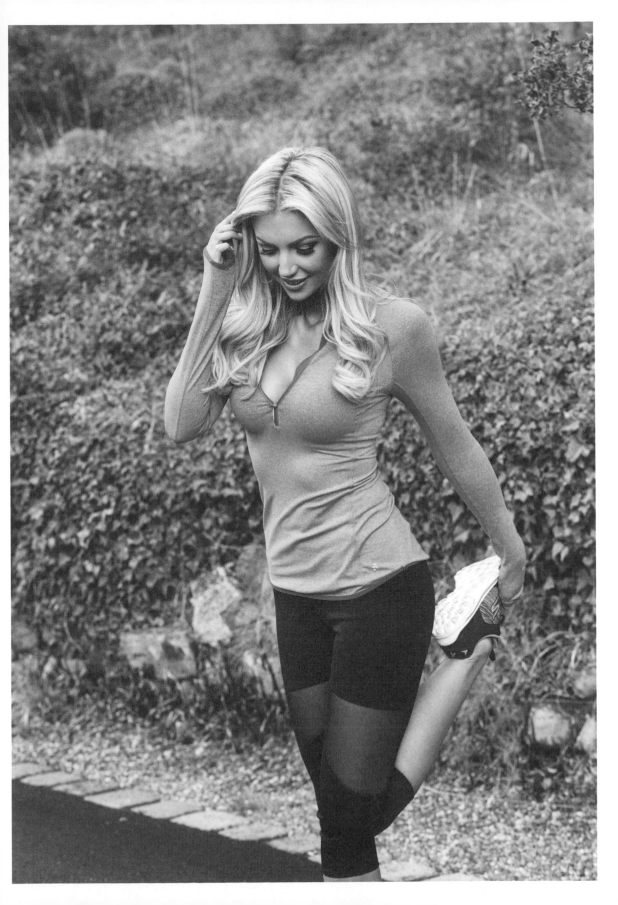

Blue Warrior Recovery Shake

SERVES 1 | PER SERVING: 212 CALORIES | 18.9G PROTEIN | 25.4G CARBS | 6.3G FAT

125ml unsweetened
almond milk

125g fresh blueberries, rinsed

1 handful of baby spinach
(optional)

1 scoop of Sunwarrior vanilla
protein powder

1 tbsp milled chia seeds
or flaxseeds

1 tsp vanilla extract or powder

4–5 drops of liquid stevia, to
sweeten (optional)

2–3 ice cubes

This smoothie is a staple for me after a challenging resistance workout, as it provides protein to repair torn muscle fibres, anti-inflammatory omega-3 fat to help soothe muscle pain and antioxidants to mop up the free radicals that are normally released during a strenuous workout. This helps to protect your cells from oxidative stress.

1   Place all the ingredients in a blender, beginning with the almond milk, and combine until smooth.
2   Serve chilled. Any leftovers can be stored in an airtight container in the fridge for two or three days.

ANTIOXIDANT-
RICH

GOOD
MOOD

LOW-
CALORIE

MUSCLE-
BUILDING

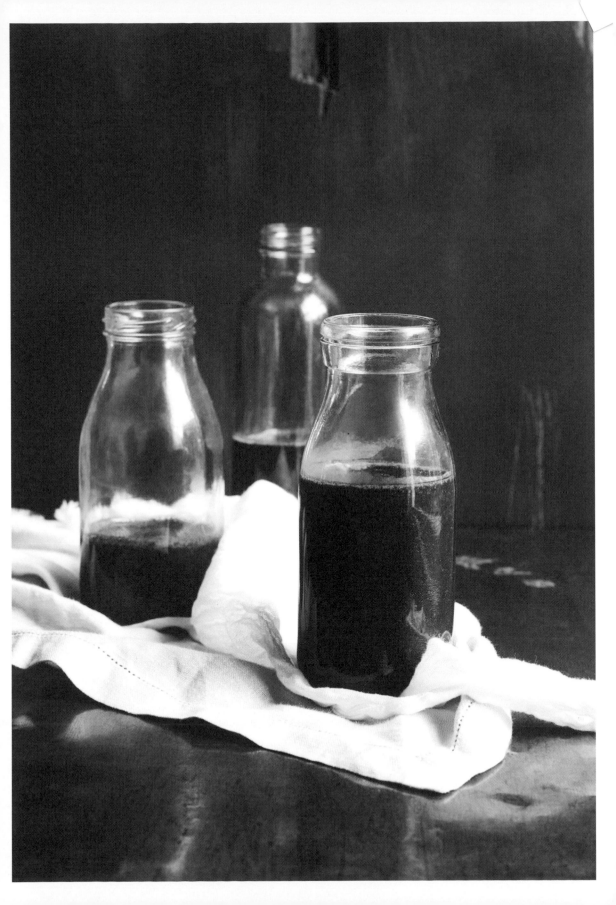

Lean Green Body Booster

SERVES 1 | PER SERVING: 197 CALORIES | 19.6G PROTEIN | 21.4G CARBS | 6G FAT

125ml unsweetened almond milk

1 large handful of baby spinach

½ banana, fresh or frozen

1 scoop of Sunwarrior vanilla protein powder

1 tsp vanilla extract or powder

1 tsp peanut butter (aim to buy an organic brand, free from added sugar and palm oil)

¾ tsp ground cinnamon

2–3 ice cubes

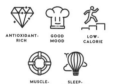

ANTIOXIDANT-RICH   GOOD MOOD   LOW-CALORIE

MUSCLE-BUILDING   SLEEP-ENHANCING

This is a great smoothie to enjoy before or after a workout or as a restorative snack at any time of the day. I often enjoy one as an afternoon pick-me-up, as it contains natural energy from the banana, the ACE antioxidant vitamins from the spinach and muscle-boosting properties from the protein and nut butter.

1   Place all the ingredients in a blender, beginning with the almond milk, and combine until smooth.
2   Serve chilled. Any leftovers can be stored in an airtight container in the fridge for up to two days.

Salted Caramel Power Smoothie

125ml unsweetened almond milk

1 ripe banana, peeled, cut into chunks and frozen for at least 2 hours

2 pitted Medjool dates or 4–5 drops of liquid stevia, to sweeten

1 scoop of Sunwarrior vanilla protein powder

1 tbsp hulled hemp seeds

1 tsp vanilla extract

pinch of sea salt

Filled with protein and fibre, this smoothie tastes delicious and fills your body with nutrients. Hemp seeds are one of the world's most perfect plant sources of the complete set of essential amino acids and they boast an ideal ratio of omega-3 to omega-6 fats. This makes them an excellent food for anyone following an active and healthy lifestyle. I enjoy this smoothie before exercise to boost my energy, or else afterwards for recovery and repair.

1   Place all the ingredients in a blender, beginning with the almond milk, and combine until smooth.

2   Serve chilled. Any leftovers can be stored in an airtight container in the fridge for up to two days.

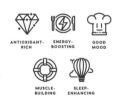

ANTIOXIDANT-RICH   ENERGY-BOOSTING   GOOD MOOD

MUSCLE-BUILDING   SLEEP-ENHANCING

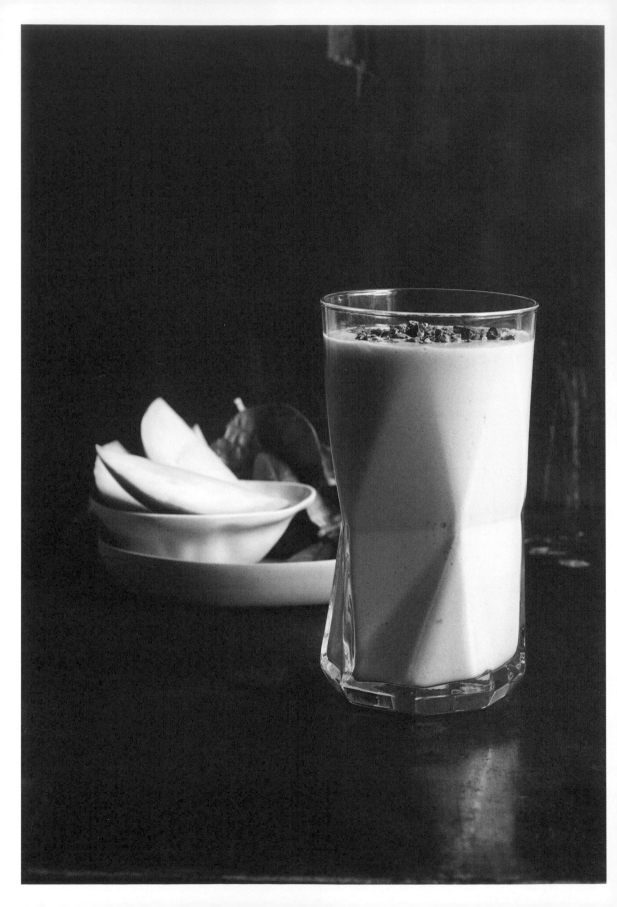

Good to Glow
Mango Tango Smoothie

SERVES 1 | PER SERVING: 205 CALORIES | 4.7G PROTEIN | 31G CARBS | 9G FAT

125ml low-fat coconut milk or unsweetened almond milk

1 large handful of baby spinach

1 small handful of fresh mint leaves

½ ripe mango, peeled, cut into chunks and frozen for 2 hours

juice of ½ lime

1 tbsp raw cashew nuts

1 tbsp unsweetened desiccated coconut, plus extra to serve

2–3 ice cubes

ANTIOXIDANT-RICH   ENERGY-BOOSTING

GOOD MOOD   SLEEP-ENHANCING

This is a deliciously cool and creamy smoothie filled with healthy fats, antioxidant vitamins and beauty minerals for a glowing complexion. Mango is one of my favourite fruits for bright and healthy skin, as it's a super source of beta-carotene, which converts to vitamin A in the body with the help of a little dietary fat. Vitamin A is then used to repair damaged skin cells.

1 Place all the ingredients in a blender, beginning with the milk, and combine until smooth and creamy.

2 Sprinkle with desiccated coconut and serve chilled. Any leftovers should stay fresh in an airtight container in the fridge for up to two days, but this smoothie is best enjoyed as soon as possible after making it.

Turmeric and Ginger Immune Booster

SERVES 1 | PER SERVING: 191 CALORIES | 2.9G PROTEIN | 44.7G CARBS | 2.2G FAT

125ml unsweetened almond milk

80g fresh pineapple chunks

1 medium carrot, peeled and roughly chopped

1 fresh or frozen banana

juice of ½ lemon or lime

1 tsp freshly grated ginger

¼ tsp ground turmeric

2–3 ice cubes

unsweetened desiccated coconut, to garnish

pomegranate seeds, to garnish

½ passionfruit, seeds scooped out, to garnish

This is a fresh, fruity smoothie with powerful anti-inflammatory properties to help soothe pain and inflammation. Turmeric and ginger have both been used medicinally for centuries. Antioxidant-rich turmeric helps to reduce inflammation and brighten the complexion, while ginger boosts blood flow, aids digestion and soothes nausea. Pineapple is similarly anti-inflammatory, banana helps to boost mood and the beta-carotene in the carrot supports healthy eyesight and a glowing complexion.

1   Place all the ingredients in a blender, beginning with the almond milk, and combine until smooth.
2   Serve chilled and garnish with a sprinkle of desiccated coconut, pomegranate seeds and passionfruit seeds. Any leftovers can be stored in an airtight container in the fridge for up to two days.

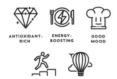

ANTIOXIDANT-RICH   ENERGY-BOOSTING   GOOD MOOD

LOW-CALORIE   SLEEP-ENHANCING

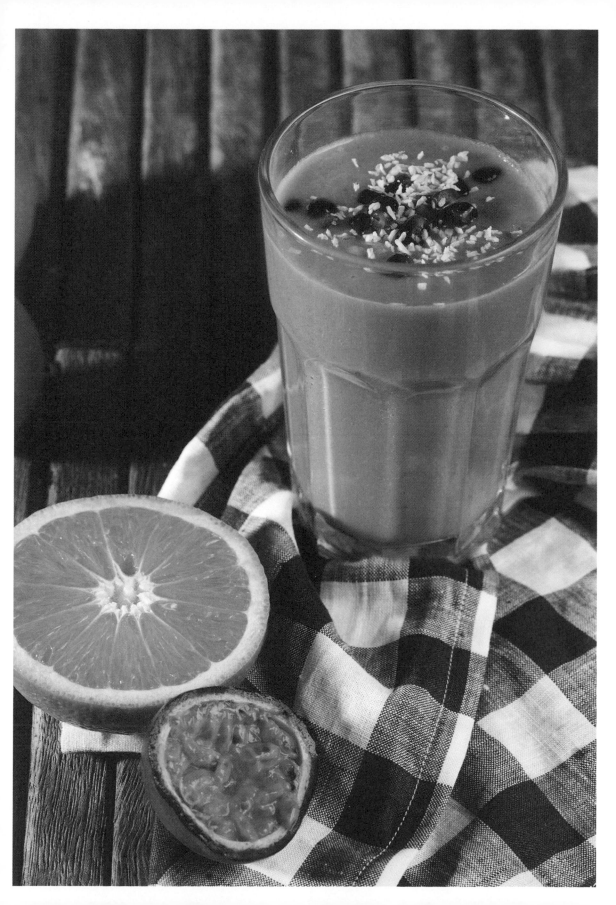

Strawberry Shortbread
Breakfast Shake

SERVES 1 | PER SERVING: 289 CALORIES | 7.4G PROTEIN | 43.7G CARBS | 11.7G FAT

125ml unsweetened
almond milk

5–6 strawberries, hulled

1 ripe fresh or frozen banana

2 heaped tbsp gluten-free
porridge oats

2 tbsp milled flaxseeds

1 tsp smooth almond butter

1 tsp ground cinnamon

1 tsp vanilla extract

4–5 drops of liquid stevia, or
to taste

3 ice cubes

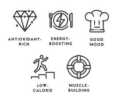

ANTIOXIDANT-
RICH   ENERGY-
BOOSTING   GOOD
MOOD

LOW-
CALORIE   MUSCLE-
BUILDING

This is a complete and nourishing breakfast in a smoothie for busy people on the go. The strawberries, banana and oats provide natural energy, antioxidants, good mood nutrients and plenty of fibre to encourage a flat stomach, while the ground flaxseeds and almond butter further boost the healthy fat and fibre content. It's designed to stabilise your blood sugar levels, which means you'll be less likely to reach for a sugary mid-morning snack.

1   Place all the ingredients in a blender, beginning with the almond milk, and combine until smooth and creamy. Add more almond milk if you prefer a runnier texture. Taste and add more cinnamon, vanilla or liquid stevia, if desired.

2   Any leftovers can be stored in an airtight container in the fridge for up to two days.

Sleepytime Almond and Cinnamon Smoothie

SERVES 1 | PER SERVING: 238 CALORIES | 4.8G PROTEIN | 41.2G CARBS | 8.5G FAT

180ml unsweetened almond milk

1 banana, peeled, cut into chunks and frozen for at least 2 hours

2–3 dates, pitted and chopped

2 tsp smooth almond butter

½ tsp ground cinnamon

2–3 ice cubes

GOOD MOOD   LOW-CALORIE   SLEEP-ENHANCING

A cool and creamy smoothie created as a sweet treat that won't impact your waistline. This shake is ideal for those evening sugar cravings and will encourage a happy, relaxed mood and a deep, restful sleep because it contains the important trio of vitamin B6, zinc and the amino acid tryptophan. Together, they enable the production of serotonin to boost your mood and melatonin to encourage good-quality sleep.

1 Place all the ingredients in a blender, beginning with the almond milk, and combine until smooth.
2 Serve chilled. Any leftovers can be stored in an airtight container in the fridge for up to two days.

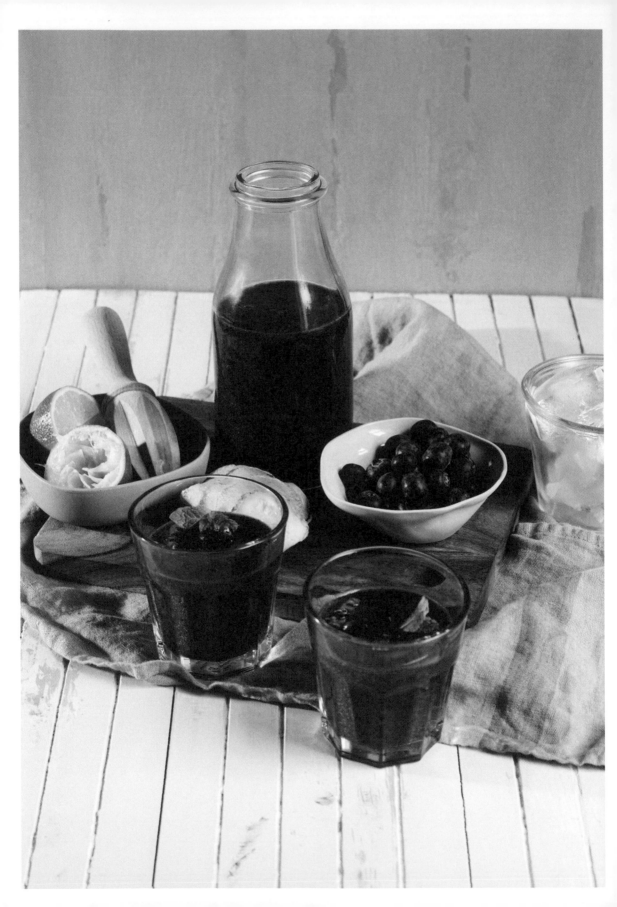

Blueberry Cleanser

SERVES 1 | PER SERVING: 210 CALORIES | 3.6G PROTEIN | 52.2G CARBS | 1.1G FAT

125ml coconut water

125g fresh or frozen
blueberries

1 ripe banana

¼ cucumber

1 small handful of fresh
mint leaves

1 small handful of fresh
flat-leaf parsley leaves

juice of ½ lime

1 tsp freshly grated ginger

3 ice cubes

4–5 drops of liquid stevia, or
to taste

ANTIOXIDANT-
RICH

GOOD
MOOD

LOW-
CALORIE

A refreshing, electrolyte-rich smoothie designed to boost kidney function, banish a bloated tummy and reduce puffiness around the eyes. Parsley is a powerful cleanser, while blueberries, banana, cucumber, ginger and coconut water work together to reduce water retention and bloating and to support healthy, normal blood pressure.

1 Place all the ingredients in a blender, starting with the coconut water, and combine until smooth. Taste and add liquid stevia if a sweeter taste is required.
2 Serve chilled. Any leftovers can be stored in a covered container in the fridge for up to two days.

Pineapple Paradise

SERVES 1 | PER SERVING: 256 CALORIES | 4.1G PROTEIN | 48.2G CARBS | 8.2G FAT

125ml chilled coconut water
or regular water

80g fresh or frozen
pineapple chunks

1 large handful of baby
spinach

1 green apple, cored and
quartered

¼ ripe avocado

¼ cucumber, cut into chunks

juice of 1 small lime

1 tsp freshly grated ginger

ANTIOXIDANT- ENERGY-
RICH   BOOSTING

LOW-
CALORIE

A healthy and refreshing green smoothie that makes a great morning or afternoon snack to boost flagging energy levels. It's a rich source of chlorophyll, which is the pigment found in green vegetables. Chlorophyll shares an almost identical structure with the haemoglobin in human red blood cells, making it an excellent blood builder and cleanser to support health and vitality.

1   Place all the ingredients in a blender, beginning with the coconut water, and combine until smooth.
2   Serve chilled. Any leftovers can be stored in an airtight container in the fridge for up to two days.

Chia Summer Berry Blast

SERVES 1 | PER SERVING: 274 CALORIES | 7G PROTEIN | 50.1G CARBS | 7.8G FAT

125ml chilled coconut water
or normal water

1 handful of baby spinach

125g fresh or frozen
blueberries

125g fresh raspberries

3–4 medium or large
strawberries, hulled

2 tbsp whole chia seeds

1 tsp vanilla extract or powder

1 tsp fresh lime juice

2–3 ice cubes

ANTIOXIDANT-
RICH

ENERGY-
BOOSTING

LOW-
CALORIE

MUSCLE-
BUILDING

Berries are an important part of my everyday diet, and I notice the difference in my skin if I don't eat them for a week or two. As one of the lowest-sugar types of fruit, berries also have one of the richest contents of antioxidants of all foods, which help to brighten your complexion. Chia seeds are one of my favourite sources of omega-3 fat for super-soft and healthy skin. I added in a handful of baby spinach for an extra dose of cleansing greens, energising iron and antioxidant vitamins A, C and E.

1 Place all the ingredients in a blender, starting with the coconut water and spinach leaves, and combine until smooth.

2 Serve chilled. Any leftovers can be stored in an airtight container in the fridge for up to two days or frozen for up to three months.

Mint Chocolate Chip Thickshake

SERVES 1 | PER SERVING (SWEETENED WITH STEVIA): 293 CALORIES | 8.4G PROTEIN

40.3G CARBS | 13.4G FAT

250ml unsweetened almond milk

1 ripe banana, peeled, cut into chunks and frozen for at least 2 hours

2 pitted Medjool dates, 1 tbsp pure maple syrup or honey or 4–5 drops of liquid stevia, to sweeten

1 small handful of fresh mint leaves or ½ tsp pure peppermint extract

2 tbsp raw cacao powder or unsweetened dark cocoa powder

1 tbsp ground flaxseeds

2 tsp smooth or crunchy almond butter

TO SERVE:

1 tsp cacao nibs or unsweetened dark chocolate chips

fresh mint leaves

fresh berries

Mint and chocolate chips are a match made in foodie heaven. This rich, creamy shake delivers a zingy blast of fresh mint and plenty of crunchy chocolate chips. Being guilt-free, healthy and nourishing makes it taste even sweeter.

1   Place all the ingredients in a blender, starting with the almond milk, and combine until smooth and creamy. Taste and add more sweetener if necessary.
2   Serve chilled, topped with cacao nibs or chocolate chips, mint leaves and berries. Any leftovers can be stored in an airtight container in the fridge for up to two days.

ANTIOXIDANT-RICH   ENERGY-BOOSTING

GOOD MOOD   SLEEP-ENHANCING

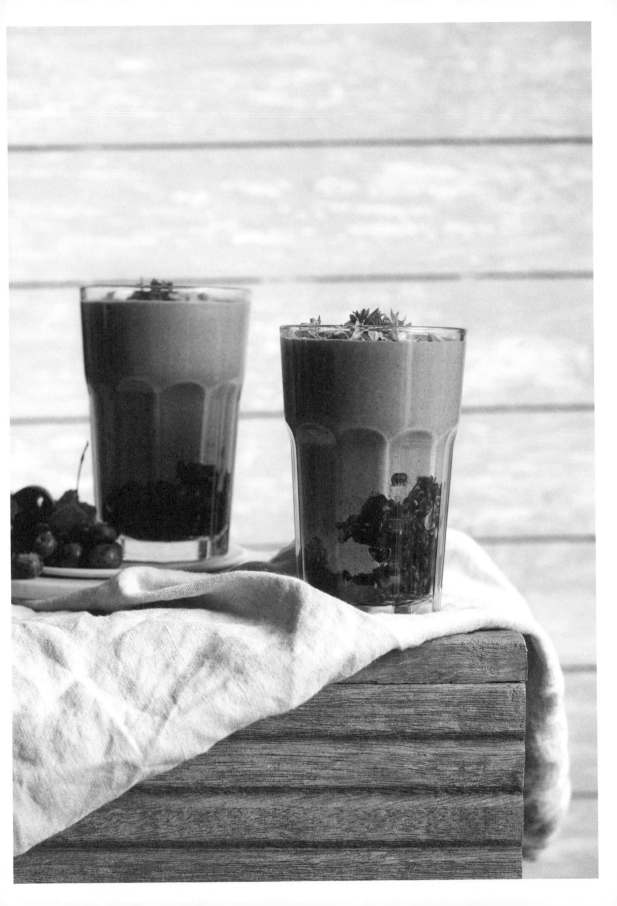

Stress-Soothing
Avocado Smoothie

SERVES 1 | PER SERVING: 224 CALORIES | 5G PROTEIN | 25.4G CARBS | 13.8G FAT

180ml unsweetened almond milk

1 handful of baby spinach

3 dates, pitted

¼ ripe avocado

1 tsp smooth unsalted almond butter

1 tsp vanilla extract

2 ice cubes

4–5 drops of liquid stevia, to taste (optional)

1 tsp whole chia seeds, to serve

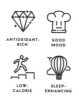

ANTIOXIDANT-RICH   GOOD MOOD

LOW-CALORIE   SLEEP-ENHANCING

Try this stress-soothing smoothie if you're having a stressful day and really need something to calm a frazzled nervous system. I designed this drink to deliver a rich dose of magnesium to every cell in your body. Magnesium is an essential driving force behind over 300 different enzyme reactions and is considered nature's most powerful relaxation mineral. Found in leafy green veggies, nuts and seeds, avocados and a vast range of other whole plant foods, it's the perfect antidote to stress, helping to relax tense muscles and even improve your sleep.

1   Place all the ingredients except the chia seeds in a blender, starting with the almond milk, and combine until smooth and creamy. Taste and add a few drops of stevia if necessary.

2   Serve chilled, garnished with chia seeds. Any leftovers can be stored in an airtight container in the fridge for up to two days.

Chocolate Peanut Butter
Protein Thickshake

SERVES 1 | PER SERVING: 191 CALORIES | 20.2G PROTEIN | 11.3G CARBS | 9G FAT

125ml unsweetened
almond milk

1 scoop of Sunwarrior
chocolate protein powder

1 tbsp raw cacao powder
or unsweetened dark cocoa
powder, plus extra to serve

2 tsp smooth or crunchy
peanut butter

1 tsp vanilla extract

2–3 ice cubes

4–5 drops of liquid stevia, to
sweeten (optional)

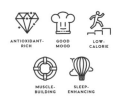

ANTIOXIDANT-RICH GOOD MOOD LOW-CALORIE

MUSCLE-BUILDING SLEEP-ENHANCING

I love this heavenly combination of decadent chocolate and peanut butter in a thick, creamy shake. Rich in protein, healthy fats and antioxidants, this smoothie is beneficial for your skin and waistline as it's free from refined sugar and empty calories. The peanut butter and protein help muscle growth and repair, while the cacao's powerful antioxidants aid in cellular protection.

1   Place all the ingredients in a blender, beginning with the almond milk, and blend until smooth and creamy. Add more almond milk if you prefer a more runny texture.

2   Serve chilled, topped with an extra pinch of cacao powder. Any leftovers can be stored in a covered container in the fridge for two or three days.

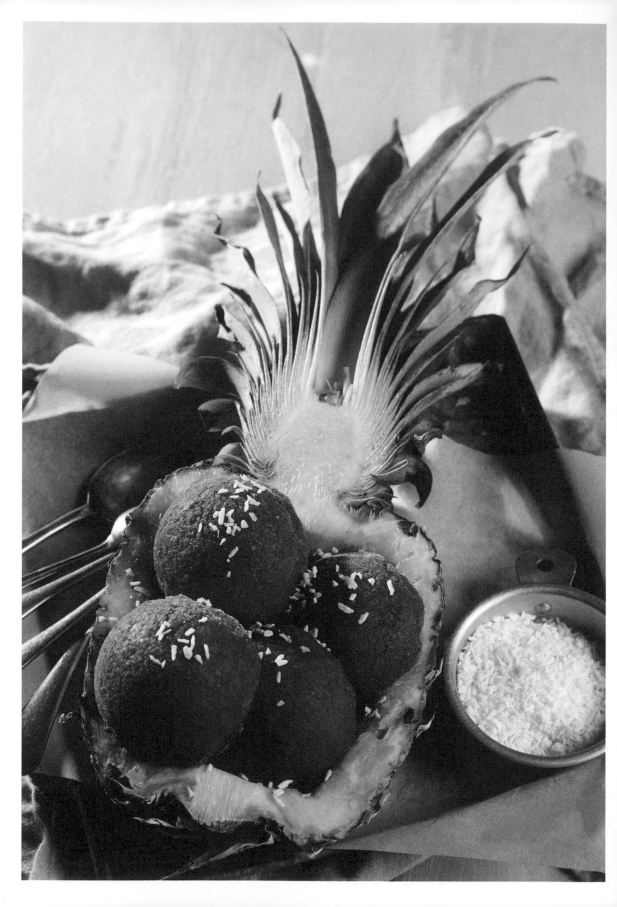

Pineapple, Raspberry and Lime Summer Sorbet

SERVES 2 | PER SERVING: 263 CALORIES | 3.3G PROTEIN | 68.5G CARBS | 0.9G FAT

1 ripe pineapple

125g fresh raspberries

1 tbsp fresh lime juice

1 tsp vanilla extract

cold water, to blend

desiccated coconut, to decorate

ANTIOXIDANT-
RICH   ENERGY-
          BOOSTING

LOW-
CALORIE

Sweet, sour, cold and refreshing, this simple, fruity sorbet is free from refined sugar and makes a delicious dessert or anytime treat. Pineapple has powerful anti-inflammatory properties, making it an ideal food to help soothe sore post-workout muscles. Pineapple also contains bromelain, which is a proteolytic enzyme. This helps to break down protein fibres, boosting digestion. Raspberries are a low-sugar fruit, full of antioxidants and fibre, and lime juice aids in cleansing the liver. I use my Vitamix blender to achieve a smooth texture. If you're not sure your blender or food processor can handle it, lightly freeze the pineapple before blending, then place it back into the freezer to set properly when blended.

1   Carefully cut the pineapple in half using a sharp serrated knife. Remove the skin from one half and cut the flesh into chunks, then place in a bowl or container. Cut the flesh out of the second half of the pineapple, leaving the skin to form a bowl for the sorbet. Add the flesh to the bowl with the pineapple chunks and place it in the freezer for at least 2 hours.

2   Place the frozen pineapple in a food processor or blender along with the raspberries, lime juice and vanilla. Use a splash of cold water to help it blend if necessary.

3   Once smooth, spoon it into the prepared pineapple half. Decorate with a sprinkle of desiccated coconut and serve immediately or place in the freezer for 20 minutes to set and then scoop into balls if you prefer.

POWER-PACKED MAINS

Fitness tip

Complete sources of PROTEIN, COMPLEX CARBS and some HEALTHY FATS are all important for building and maintaining lean muscle, reducing body fat and sustaining ENERGY LEVELS. Every one of these power-packed mains, soups and salads is designed to boost vitality and support and improve fitness levels and body composition, depending on your personal goals. Some are LOW-CALORIE and some are more hearty, but all are packed with DELICIOUS FLAVOURS, simple to make and created to help you reach your highest HEALTH and FITNESS POTENTIAL.

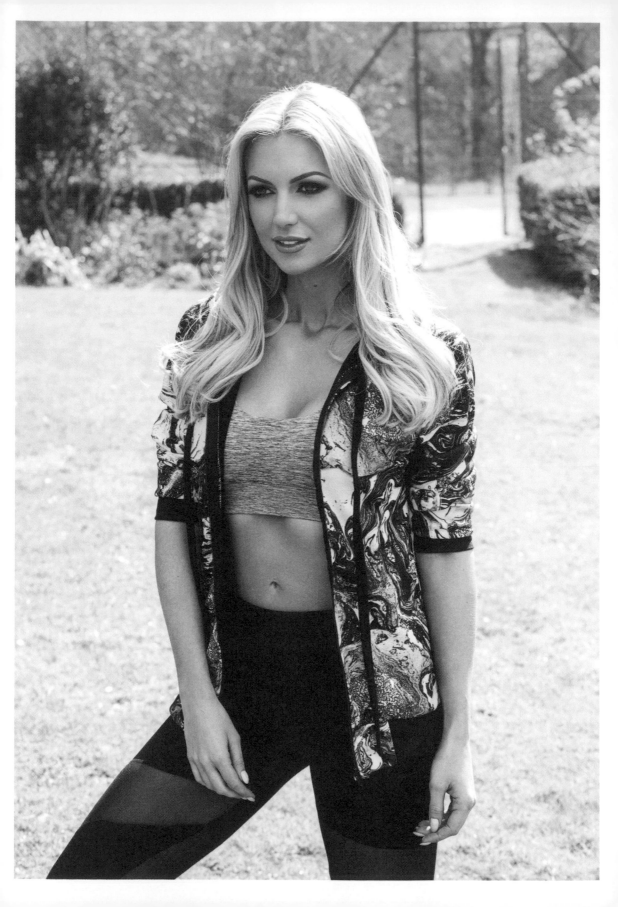

Lean Green Soup

SERVES 5–6 | PER SERVING: 74 CALORIES | 4.3G PROTEIN | 13G CARBS | 1.3G FAT

2 tbsp low-sodium tamari or water

1 red onion, finely diced

3 garlic cloves, minced

1 tsp finely chopped fresh ginger

3 courgettes, sliced

200g fine green beans, chopped

200g frozen peas

135g broccoli florets

1.2 litres low-sodium vegetable stock

3 tbsp fresh mint leaves

1 tsp dried thyme

pinch of dried chilli flakes (optional)

sea salt and freshly ground black pepper

ANTIOXIDANT-RICH   ENERGY-BOOSTING

LOW-CALORIE

Green smoothies are a wonderful addition to your diet in warmer months, but when your body craves hot food in wintertime, this soup is perfect for boosting your intake of greens and increasing your energy levels too. Filling and rich in fibre yet low in calories, it's ideal for making in a big batch and enjoying over a few days. I love it with a slice of the toasted roast garlic and rosemary bread on page 226.

1   Heat the tamari or water in a large saucepan set over a medium heat, then add the onion, garlic and ginger and cook for 4–5 minutes, until the onions have softened. Add the courgettes, green beans, peas and broccoli and cook for 3–4 minutes, stirring well. Add the stock, mint, thyme, chilli flakes, if using, and some seasoning. Bring it to the boil for 3–4 minutes, then lower the heat and allow the vegetables to simmer for 25–30 minutes, until soft.

2   Transfer the soup to a blender or else use a hand-held blender to blitz the soup until smooth. Taste and adjust the seasoning if necessary. Serve hot. Any leftovers can be stored in an airtight container in the fridge for three or four days or frozen for up to three months.

Carrot, Coconut and Red Lentil Soup

SERVES 2 | PER SERVING: 266 CALORIES | 12G PROTEIN | 50G CARBS | 3.3G FAT

2 tbsp low-sodium tamari or water

1 red onion, finely chopped

2 garlic cloves, minced

1 tbsp finely chopped or grated fresh ginger

8 medium carrots, cut into chunks

2 celery stalks, cut into chunks

2 tsp chopped fresh thyme or 1 tsp dried thyme

500ml low-sodium vegetable stock

250ml low-fat coconut milk

4 tbsp split red lentils

1 tbsp fresh lemon juice

2 tsp smoked paprika

1 tsp ground turmeric

sea salt and freshly ground black pepper

2 tsp unsweetened desiccated coconut, to garnish

Carrot and coconut work deliciously well to produce a smooth, creamy texture, while the split red lentils add a blast of high-fibre protein for a soup that will keep you feeling full for hours.

1   In a large saucepan set over a medium-high heat, heat up the tamari or water. Add the onion, garlic and ginger and cook for 4–5 minutes, until the onion begins to soften. Add the carrots, celery and thyme and cook for 5–6 minutes, until the carrots begin to soften, stirring frequently.

2   Add the vegetable stock, coconut milk, lentils, lemon juice, smoked paprika, turmeric and salt and pepper to taste. Ensure that the vegetables are fully covered in the liquid, then partly cover the saucepan with a lid, turn the heat up and bring to the boil for 2–3 minutes. Bring the heat down to medium and allow the soup to simmer for 15–20 minutes, until the carrots are soft and the lentils are cooked through.

3   Transfer the soup to a blender and blitz on high power until the soup is smooth and creamy, or use a hand-held soup blender to blend it in the saucepan. Serve hot, topped with a sprinkle of desiccated coconut. Any leftovers can be stored in a covered container in the fridge for three or four days.

ANTIOXIDANT-RICH   LOW-CALORIE

MUSCLE-BUILDING

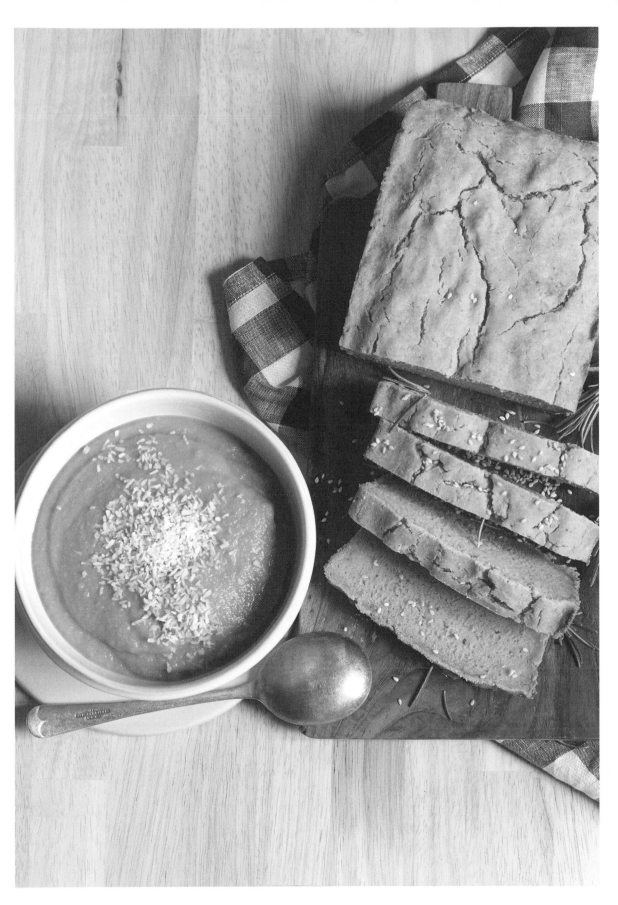

Curried Cauliflower and Sweet Potato Soup

SERVES 4 | PER SERVING: 126 CALORIES | 6.1G PROTEIN | 26.8G CARBS | 0.8G FAT

coconut oil, to grease

1 head of cauliflower, cut into florets

2 medium sweet potatoes, peeled and cut into chunks

2 garlic cloves, peeled

sea salt and freshly ground black pepper

3 tbsp tamari

1 red onion, finely sliced

1 tbsp curry powder

2 tsp finely chopped fresh ginger

750ml low-sodium vegetable stock

1 tsp ground turmeric

pinch of cayenne pepper (optional)

2 tbsp chopped fresh coriander, to garnish

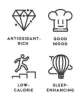

ANTIOXIDANT-RICH   GOOD MOOD

LOW-CALORIE   SLEEP-ENHANCING

Cauliflower and curry spices make a delicious duo and work perfectly with the caramelised sweetness of roast sweet potato and garlic. This is my idea of a perfect lunch.

1 Preheat the oven to 190°C. Lightly grease a large baking tray with coconut oil or line with non-stick baking paper.

2 Spread out the cauliflower florets, sweet potato chunks and garlic cloves on the lined tray and lightly season with sea salt and black pepper. Place the tray in the oven and roast the vegetables for 30–35 minutes, until lightly golden and crisp. Set aside.

3 Heat up the tamari in a large saucepan set over a medium heat. Sauté the onion for 2–3 minutes, until it begins to soften, then add the curry powder and ginger and continue to stir for another 1–2 minutes. Add the vegetable stock to the saucepan, followed by the roast cauliflower, sweet potato and garlic, then stir in the turmeric, cayenne pepper, if using, and some salt and pepper. Bring the soup to the boil for 2–3 minutes, then cover partly with a lid, lower the heat and allow it to simmer gently for about 10 minutes.

4 Transfer the soup to a blender and blend on high until smooth, or keep it in the saucepan and use a hand-held blender to blend the ingredients into a soup. Serve hot garnished with the chopped fresh coriander. Any leftovers can be stored in a covered container in the fridge for up to four days.

Skinny Cauliflower Tabbouleh with Toasted Sesame Seeds

SERVES 4 | PER SERVING: 66 CALORIES | 1.7G PROTEIN | 8.3G CARBS | 3.6G FAT

4 tbsp sesame seeds

500g cauliflower

60g fresh flat-leaf parsley, chopped

20g fresh mint leaves, chopped

1 red onion, finely chopped

1 garlic clove, minced

15 cherry tomatoes, quartered

10–12 pitted Kalamata or other black olives (optional)

¼ cucumber, chopped into cubes

2 tbsp fresh lemon juice

2 tbsp tamari

2 tsp cold-pressed extra virgin olive oil

1 tsp smoked paprika

pinch of dried chilli flakes (optional)

sea salt and freshly ground black pepper

ANTIOXIDANT-RICH   LOW-CALORIE

This version of tabbouleh contains all the familiar flavours of the traditional dish, including plenty of parsley, but uses finely processed cauliflower to make it a lighter alternative.

1 Preheat the oven to 180°C.
2 Spread out the sesame seeds on a small tray. Toast for 10–12 minutes, until golden. Remove from the oven and set aside.
3 Rinse the cauliflower and cut into chunks. Place it in a food processor and pulse until it becomes like coarse grains, similar to couscous. Transfer to a large mixing bowl and add the remaining ingredients.
4 Top with the toasted sesame seeds and serve chilled. Any leftovers can be stored in an airtight container in the fridge for three or four days.

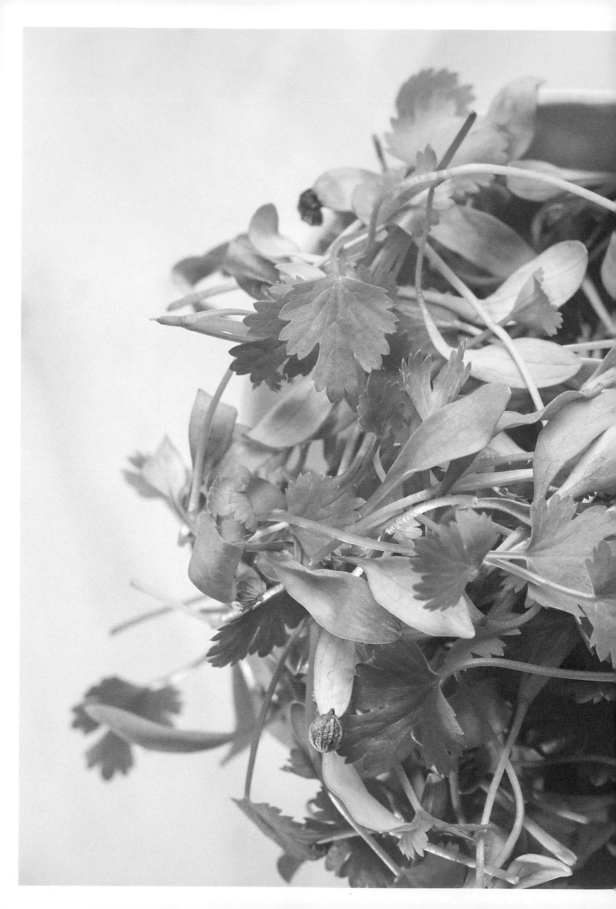

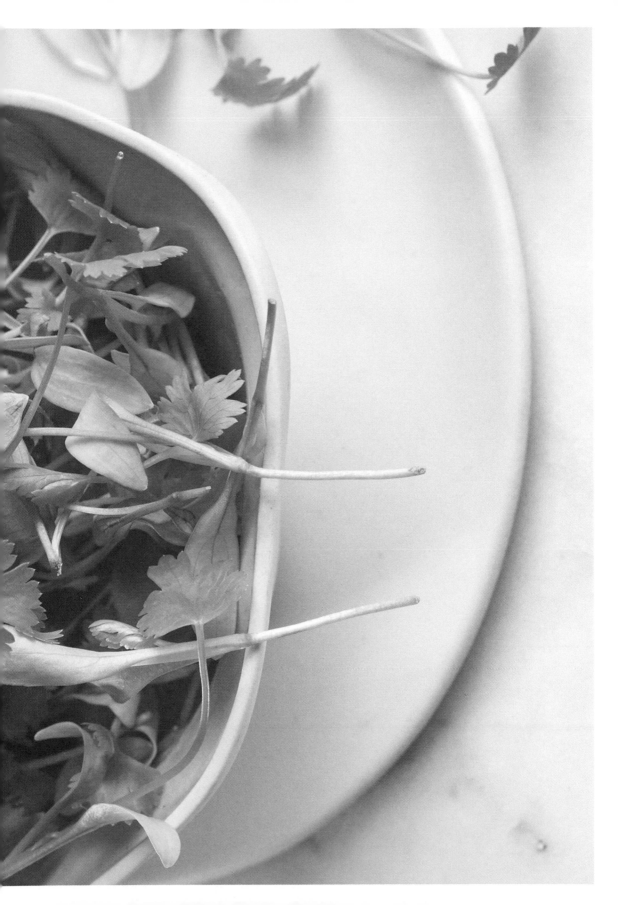

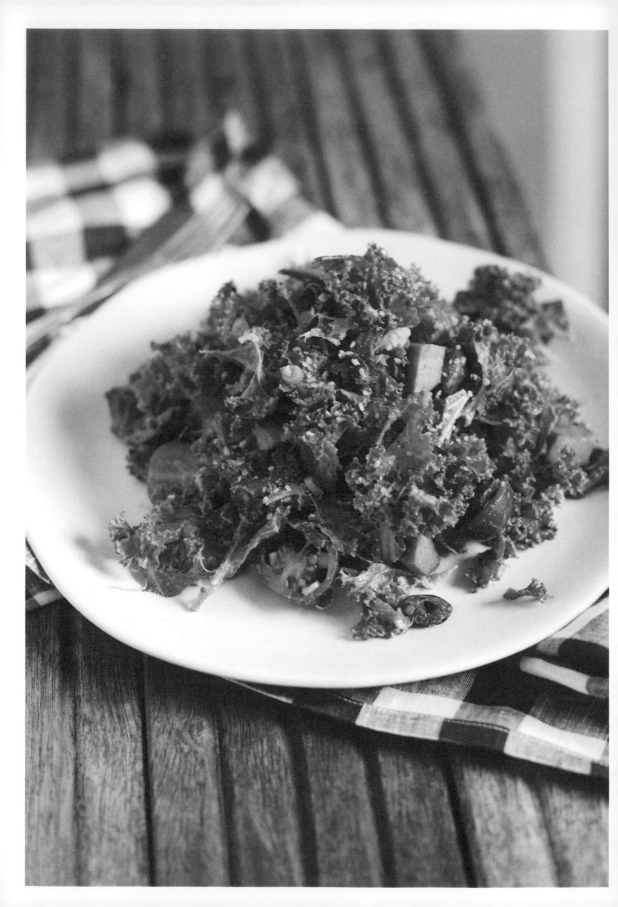

The Ultimate Kale Salad

SERVES 2 | PER SERVING: 434 CALORIES | 20G PROTEIN | 47.6G CARBS | 22.8G FAT

coconut oil, to grease

1 medium sweet potato, peeled and cut into bite-sized chunks

3 tbsp tamari

½ tsp smoked paprika

200g fresh kale

1 ripe avocado

4 tbsp nutritional yeast (optional but advised)

2 tbsp fresh lemon juice

sea salt and freshly ground black pepper

10–12 cherry tomatoes, halved

10–12 Kalamata or other black olives, pitted

4 spring onions, chopped

pinch of dried chilli flakes (optional)

2 tbsp hulled hemp seeds

ANTIOXIDANT-RICH   LOW-CALORIE

MUSCLE-BUILDING

A hearty, wholesome and satisfying kale salad, this is one of my absolute favourite go-to healthy meals. Massaging the avocado, lemon juice and sea salt into the kale helps to break down its waxy leaves and gives a delicious taste and texture to the salad.

1   Preheat the oven to 200°C. Lightly grease a baking tray with coconut oil or line non-stick baking paper.

2   Spread the sweet potato chunks out on the tray. Drizzle with 1 tablespoon of the tamari, then sprinkle on the smoked paprika. Roast in the oven for 20–25 minutes, until golden brown and crisp. Set aside.

3   Wash the kale well and pat dry. Remove the tough stems, then tear the leaves into smaller pieces and place in a large mixing bowl.

4   Cut the avocado in half, remove the stone and scoop out the flesh into the mixing bowl. Add the nutritional yeast, lemon juice and a pinch of salt and pepper. Using your hands, massage the mixture into the kale leaves until they become tender and well coated, then top with the roast sweet potato, cherry tomatoes, olives, spring onions and chilli flakes, if using. Drizzle on the remaining 2 tablespoons of tamari and mix everything together well.

5   Divide into serving bowls, top with hemp seeds and serve. Any leftovers can be stored in an airtight container in the fridge for up to three days.

Carrot Noodle Salad with Ginger-Miso Dressing

SERVES 2 | PER SERVING: 204 CALORIES | 5.4G PROTEIN | 17.9G CARBS | 14.4G FAT

1 tbsp sesame seeds

2 large carrots

1 courgette

1 cucumber

½ ripe avocado, stoned,
halved and cut into cubes

4 spring onions,
finely chopped

2 handfuls of fresh coriander,
chopped

**FOR THE GINGER-MISO
DRESSING:**

juice of ½ fresh lime

3 tbsp cold water

1 tbsp tahini

1 tsp miso paste

½ tsp chopped fresh ginger

½ tsp smoked paprika

½ tsp Japanese ume
plum seasoning

sea salt and freshly ground
black pepper

ANTIOXIDANT-
RICH

LOW-
CALORIE

Crisp and creamy, this nutritious salad makes a great light meal drizzled with a tangy ginger-miso dressing and topped with crunchy sesame seeds.

1   Preheat the oven to 190°C.
2   Spread the sesame seeds on a small tray. Toast in the oven for 8–10 minutes, until lightly browned. Allow to cool while you prepare the rest of the salad.
3   Prepare the carrot, courgette and cucumber noodles using a spiraliser or vegetable peeler and place in a large mixing bowl. Add the avocado, spring onions and coriander and mix well.
4   Place all the ginger-miso dressing ingredients in a blender or food processor and blitz until smooth and creamy. Taste and season as needed. Pour the dressing over the vegetables and toss them in the dressing.
5   Divide the salad between two bowls and top with the toasted sesame seeds.

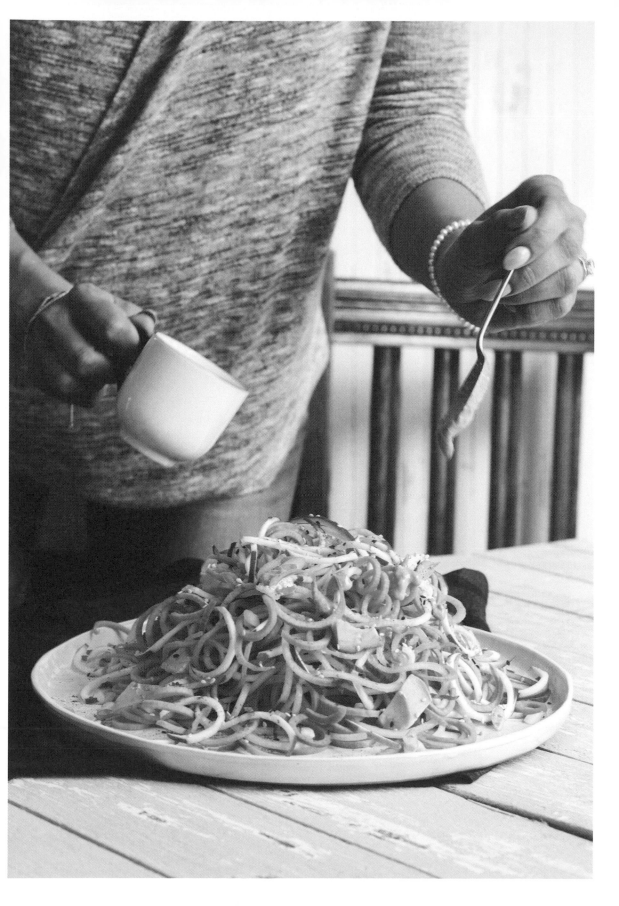

Ginger, Chilli and Lime Broccoli with Toasted Sesame Seeds

SERVES 2 | PER SERVING: 65 CALORIES | 3.1G PROTEIN | 10G CARBS | 2.6G FAT

1 tbsp sesame seeds

1 head of broccoli, broken into florets

1 garlic clove, minced

¼ red chilli, deseeded and finely chopped

1 tbsp tamari

1 tbsp fresh lime juice

1 tsp finely chopped or grated fresh ginger

sea salt and freshly ground black pepper

ANTIOXIDANT-RICH   LOW-CALORIE

This is one of the best ways to dress up steamed broccoli and turn it into a really tasty little side dish or as part of your main meal. As a filling and fibre-rich but low-calorie, low-carb vegetable, broccoli is a great food for anyone on a mission to lose a few pounds of body fat.

1   Preheat the oven to 190°C.
2   Spread the sesame seeds out on a small baking tray. Toast in the oven for 10–12 minutes, until golden, then set aside.
3   Half fill a medium-sized saucepan with cold water and top with a steamer basket or colander to steam the broccoli. Heat the water over a medium-high temperature until the water starts to simmer, then spread the broccoli evenly across the basket and cover with a lid. Steam the broccoli for just 4–5 minutes, until it has softened but remains quite crunchy.
4   Transfer the broccoli to a mixing bowl and add the garlic, chilli, tamari, lime juice, ginger, toasted sesame seeds and some salt and pepper. Toss all the ingredients together well and serve.
5   Any leftovers can be stored in an airtight container in the fridge for up to three days.

Sweet Potato and Avocado Bruschetta with Smoky Red Pepper Hummus

SERVES 2 | PER SERVING: 536 CALORIES | 11.4G PROTEIN | 51.3G CARBS | 25.2G FAT

coconut oil, to grease

2 medium sweet potatoes

1 tbsp tamari

1 tsp smoked paprika

sea salt and freshly ground black pepper

1 ripe avocado, halved, stoned and thinly sliced

1 yellow or red bell pepper, deseeded and finely sliced

2 spring onions, thinly sliced

1 handful of fresh coriander, chopped

FOR THE SMOKY RED PEPPER HUMMUS:

50g raw walnuts, chopped

2 large red bell peppers, deseeded and roughly chopped

1 garlic clove, chopped

2–4 tbsp unsweetened almond milk, to blend

1 tsp smoked paprika

pinch of cayenne pepper (optional)

ANTIOXIDANT-RICH · GOOD MOOD · MUSCLE-BUILDING · SLEEP-ENHANCING

The Italian favourite just got a whole lot healthier with my crisp, roasted sweet potato version of bruschetta. Normally made using bread, the slices of sweet potato are more filling and nutritious, topped with a thick spread of smoky red pepper hummus and chopped veggies.

1   Preheat the oven to 200°C. Lightly grease a baking tray with coconut oil or line with a sheet of non-stick baking paper.

2   Peel the sweet potatoes and use a sharp serrated knife to slice each of them lengthways into three slices (make it four slices if you prefer them thinner). Lay out the slices on the baking tray, drizzle with the tamari and sprinkle with smoked paprika and some salt and pepper to taste. Bake the potatoes in the oven for 20–25 minutes, until they turn golden brown and crisp around the edges. Remove from the heat and set aside.

3   To make the hummus, place all the ingredients in a food processor or blender. If you think your machine will have trouble blending the walnuts, soak them first in a bowl of cold water for 1–2 hours. Blend on a high speed until the mixture is smooth, using extra almond milk or water to help it blend if necessary. Season to taste with salt and pepper.

4   Spread the hummus on top of the sweet potato bruschetta, then top with some avocado, pepper, spring onions and coriander. Season again as needed. Any leftovers can be stored in an airtight container in the fridge for two or three days.

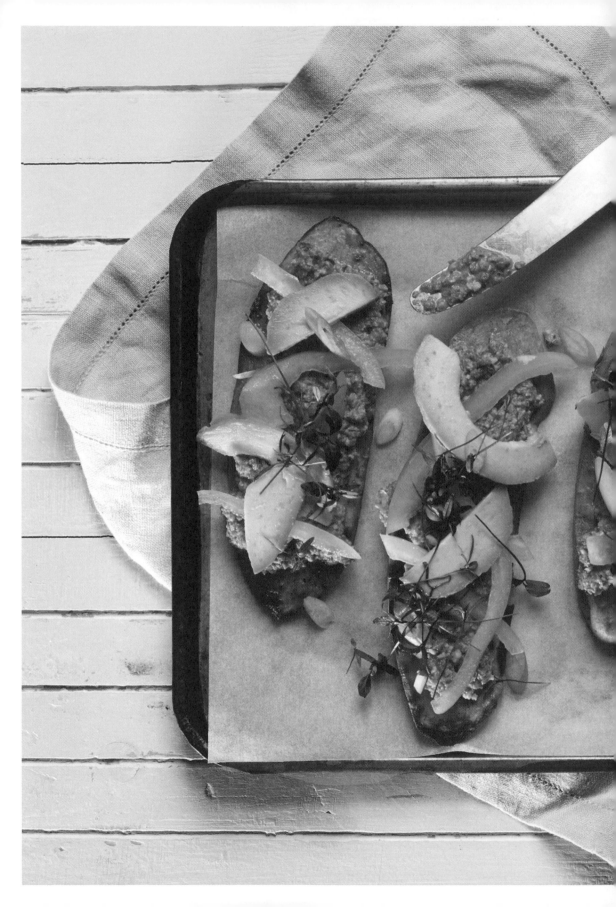

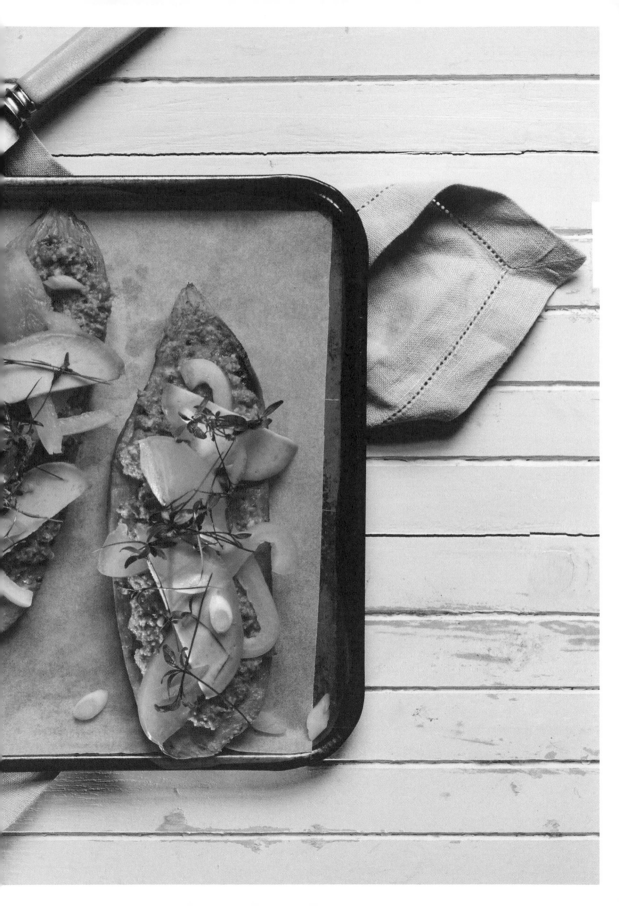

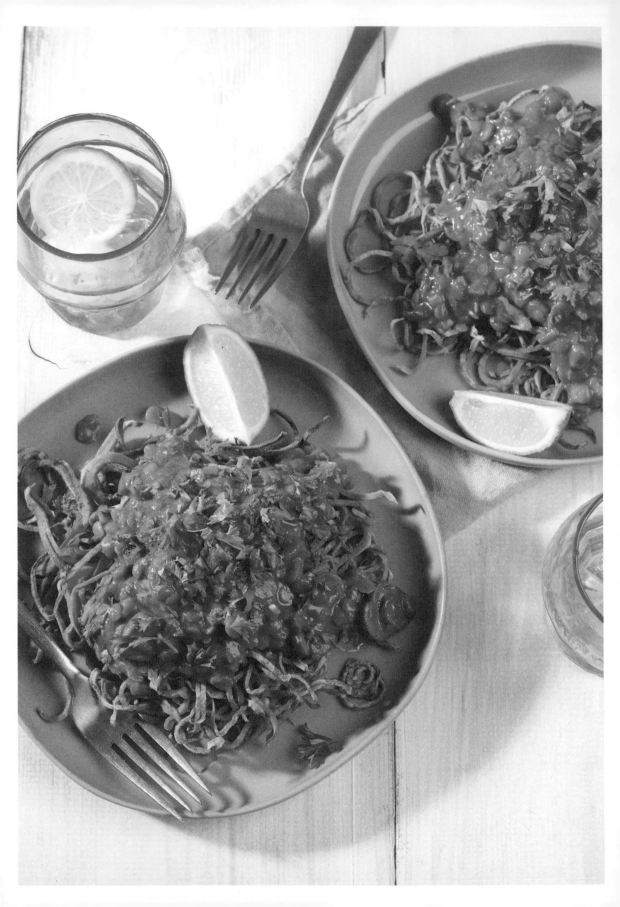

Baked Sweet Potato Noodles with Red and Yellow Dahl

SERVES 2 | PER SERVING: 385 CALORIES | 27.2G PROTEIN | 43G CARBS | 14.8G FAT

FOR THE BAKED SWEET POTATO NOODLES:

coconut oil, to grease

1 large or 2 medium sweet potatoes

1 tsp smoked paprika

sea salt and freshly ground black pepper

FOR THE LENTIL DAHL:

2 tbsp low-sodium tamari or water

1 small or medium red onion, diced

1 garlic clove, minced

1 tsp chopped fresh ginger

625ml low-fat coconut milk

4 tbsp tomato purée

2 tsp smoked paprika

1 tsp ground turmeric

1 tsp ground coriander

pinch of dried chilli flakes

95g white mushrooms, sliced

90g split yellow peas

90g split red lentils

1 handful of fresh parsley, chopped, to serve

lime wedges, to serve

Baked sweet potato noodles are one of my favourite meals because they're so healthy, versatile and can be prepared with many different flavours. I've paired them here with a protein- and fibre-rich coconut milk dahl made with red lentils and split yellow peas for a really nourishing yet low-calorie meal.

1   Preheat the oven to 190°C. Lightly grease a baking tray with coconut oil or line it with a sheet of non-stick baking paper.

2   Peel the sweet potato and cut off the pointed ends. Process the sweet potato through a spiraliser or vegetable peeler to create noodles. Spread the noodles out on the tray and sprinkle with the smoked paprika and salt and pepper to taste.

3   Bake the noodles for 15–20 minutes, until they begin to turn golden brown. Toss them with a fork halfway through the baking time to turn them over. When baked, remove the tray from the oven and set aside.

4   In a saucepan set over a medium heat, heat up the tamari or water and cook the onion, garlic and ginger for 3–4 minutes, until they soften. Add the coconut milk, tomato purée, spices and seasoning and mix well, then add the mushrooms, split peas and lentils. Partly cover the saucepan with a lid and allow the mixture to simmer for 15–20 minutes, stirring regularly to ensure it doesn't burn. Remove the lid for the final few minutes to allow any liquid to evaporate more quickly, or else add some warm water if it appears too thick. Taste at this point and adjust the seasoning if necessary.

5   Serve the noodles topped with the lentil dahl. Sprinkle with the chopped parsley and place some lime wedges on the side.

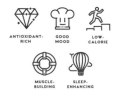

ANTIOXIDANT-RICH   GOOD MOOD   LOW-CALORIE

MUSCLE-BUILDING   SLEEP-ENHANCING

Coconut, Chickpea, Spinach and Sun-Dried Tomato Stew

SERVES 4 | PER SERVING (WITH QUINOA): 339 CALORIES | 15.6G PROTEIN | 57.3G CARBS | 8G FAT

2 tbsp low-sodium tamari or water

1 small red onion, finely chopped

55g sun-dried tomatoes, chopped

4 garlic cloves, minced

1 tbsp grated fresh ginger

zest of 1 lemon

pinch of dried chilli flakes (optional)

1 x 400g tin of cooked chickpeas, drained and rinsed

200g baby spinach

1 x 400ml tin of low-fat coconut milk, shaken well before opening

2 tbsp fresh lemon juice

2 tsp smoked paprika

1 tsp ground turmeric

sea salt and freshly ground black pepper

180g quinoa

chopped fresh coriander, to garnish

unsweetened desiccated coconut, to garnish

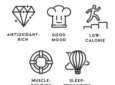

ANTIOXIDANT-RICH   GOOD MOOD   LOW-CALORIE

MUSCLE-BUILDING   SLEEP-ENHANCING

Chickpeas, spinach and sun-dried tomatoes are three of my favourite foods, so it made sense to gather them all into one deliciously warming stew. This is a great meal to make in a big batch at the beginning of the week and eat over a few days. Enjoy it with a side of fluffy quinoa for a nourishing, low-fat and high-protein meal.

1   In a large saucepan set over a medium-high heat, heat up the tamari or water. Add the onion and cook for about 5 minutes, until the onion starts to soften. Add the sun-dried tomatoes, garlic, ginger, lemon zest and chilli flakes, if using. Cook for 3 minutes, stirring frequently to prevent them from burning.

2   Turn the heat up to high and add the chickpeas. Cook for 2–3 minutes, until they're coated with the garlic, ginger and onion mixture and are beginning to turn golden. Add the spinach to the saucepan one handful at a time, stirring to allow it to wilt. Pour in the coconut milk and add the lemon juice, smoked paprika, ground turmeric, salt and pepper. Bring the stew to a simmer, then turn down the heat and cook for 10 minutes, until the chickpeas are warmed through. Taste and add more salt and lemon juice, if desired.

3   Meanwhile, to cook the quinoa, first rinse it well in a sieve under cold running water. Place the rinsed quinoa in a medium-sized saucepan and cover with double its volume of water. Cover the saucepan partly with the lid and bring it to the boil for 2–3 minutes, then lower the heat and allow it to simmer for 10–12 minutes, until most of the water has evaporated and the quinoa seeds have opened out. Remove from the heat and set aside to absorb the remaining water. Season with a pinch of sea salt and freshly ground black pepper.

4   When you're ready to serve, use a fork to fluff up the quinoa. Divide the quinoa between four bowls and top with the stew. Garnish with the chopped coriander and unsweetened desiccated coconut.

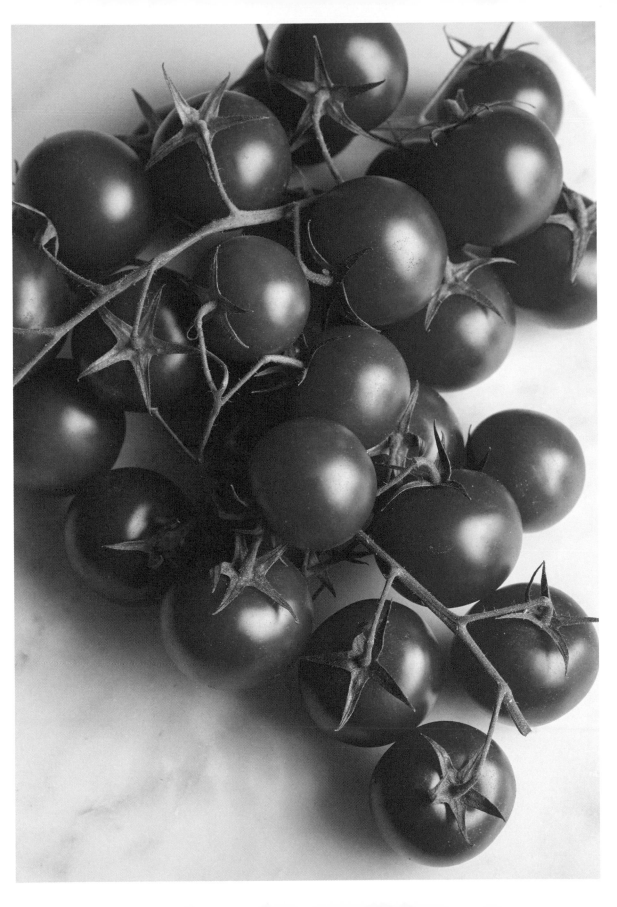

Creamy Mushroom and Quinoa Stroganoff

SERVES 2 | PER SERVING: 286 CALORIES | 27.6G PROTEIN | 56.2G CARBS | 16.4G FAT

2 tbsp low-sodium tamari
or water

1 red onion, finely chopped

2 garlic cloves, minced

500g sliced Portobello or
white mushrooms, chopped

125ml low-sodium
vegetable stock

2 tbsp low-fat coconut milk

1 tbsp fresh lemon juice

3 tbsp nutritional yeast

1½ tsp smoked paprika

1 tsp Dijon mustard

pinch of cayenne pepper

sea salt and freshly ground
black pepper

1 handful of fresh parsley,
finely chopped, plus extra
to garnish

90g quinoa

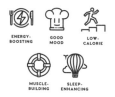

ENERGY-
BOOSTING   GOOD
MOOD   LOW-
CALORIE

MUSCLE-
BUILDING   SLEEP-
ENHANCING

This is one of my favourite hearty and healthy comfort food meals, perfect for those that crave a 'meatier' texture. Made with chunky mushrooms and a smooth and creamy herbed sauce, it's rich in flavour and super satisfying served with quinoa.

1   Heat the tamari or water in a large saucepan and add the onion and garlic. Cook for 4–5 minutes, until the onion softens. Add the mushrooms and cook for another 8–10 minutes, until lightly browned. Add the vegetable stock, coconut milk and lemon juice, then stir in the nutritional yeast, smoked paprika, mustard, cayenne pepper and seasoning. Partly cover the saucepan and simmer for 5–6 minutes. Lower the heat, remove the lid and stir the mixture, allowing any excess liquid to evaporate. Add the parsley, stir well and adjust the seasoning as needed. Remove from the heat and set aside.

2   To cook the quinoa, first rinse it well under cold running water. Place the quinoa into a medium-sized saucepan and cover with double its volume of water. Cover the saucepan partly with the lid and bring it to the boil for 2–3 minutes, then lower the heat and allow it to simmer for 10–12 minutes, until most of the water has evaporated and the quinoa seeds have opened out. Remove from the heat and set it aside to absorb the remaining water. Season with a pinch of sea salt and freshly ground black pepper.

3   To serve, use a fork to fluff up the quinoa. Divide it between two bowls or plates and serve the mushroom stroganoff on top, garnished with fresh parsley. Any leftovers can be stored in a covered container in the fridge for two or three days.

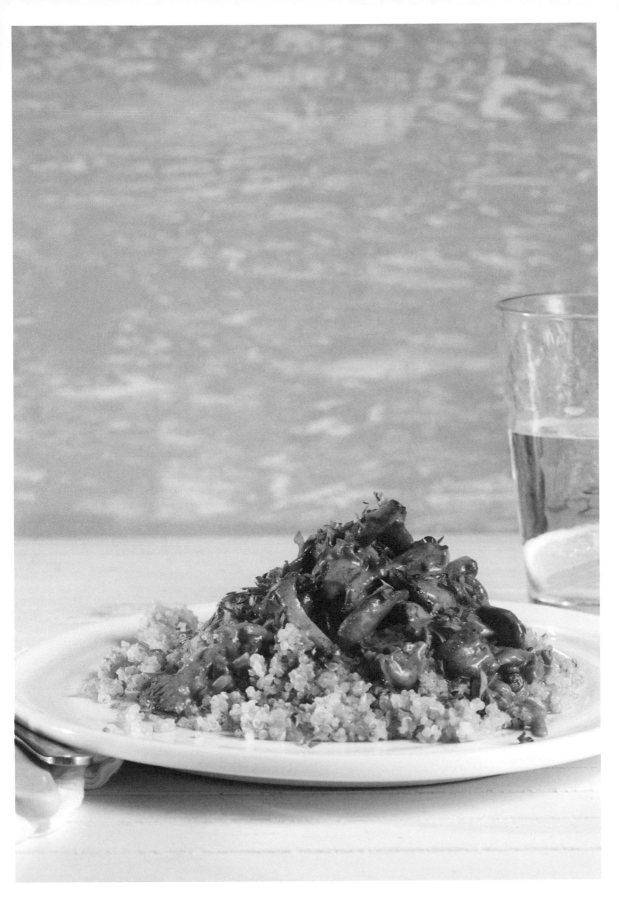

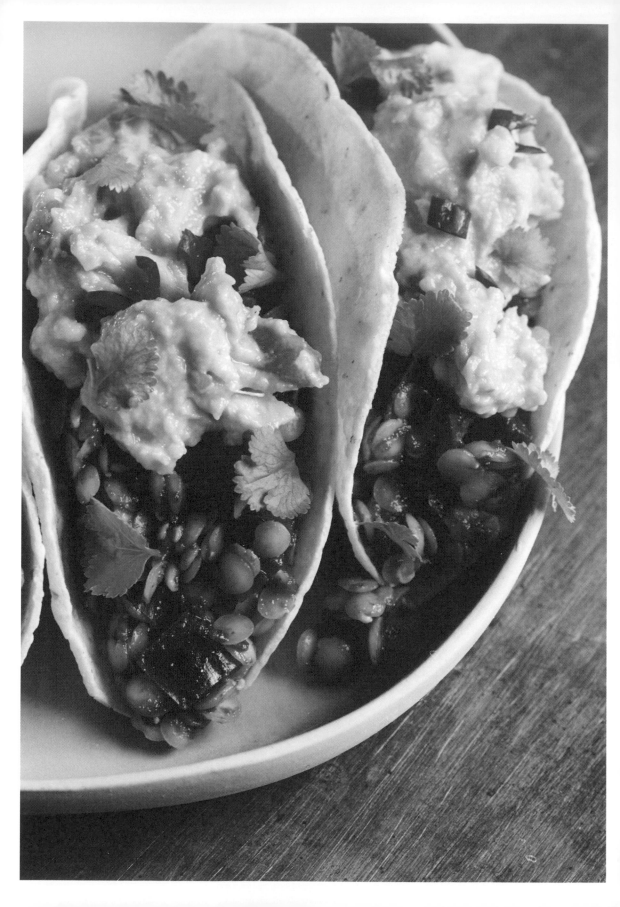

Lime and Chilli Red Lentil Tacos with Guacamole

SERVES 4 | PER SERVING (WITH GUACAMOLE): 357 CALORIES | 13.8G PROTEIN | 28G CARBS | 8.2G FAT

500ml water

200g split red lentils

2 tbsp low-sodium tamari or water

1 red onion, finely chopped

2 garlic cloves, minced

2 tbsp tomato purée

1 tsp smoked paprika

½ tsp ground cumin

zest and juice of 1 lime

pinch of dried chilli flakes (optional)

sea salt and freshly ground black pepper

tortilla wraps, taco shells or 2 heads of iceberg lettuce, to serve

fresh coriander leaves, to garnish

FOR THE GUACAMOLE:

2 ripe avocados, halved and pitted

2 medium tomatoes

2 garlic cloves, peeled

2 tbsp fresh lemon juice

1 tsp smoked paprika

pinch of cayenne pepper (optional)

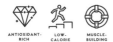

ANTIOXIDANT-RICH   LOW-CALORIE   MUSCLE-BUILDING

Lentils are one of the best foods for keeping body fat low and building lean muscle. As a complete protein, they contain all the essential amino acids plus fibre, minerals and antioxidants. I love split red lentils as they're easy and quick to cook, and they taste great mixed with spices and served with guacamole. Avocado helps to build smooth, firm, plump skin and it quenches dehydrated skin with plenty of essential fatty acids. The vitamin C in the lemon boosts collagen production for a younger-looking complexion.

1   Heat the water in a medium saucepan set over a medium-high heat and add the dried lentils. Bring the water up to the boil for 2–3 minutes, then lower the heat, partly cover the saucepan with a lid and simmer for 15–20 minutes, until the lentils are soft and cooked through. Remove from the heat and drain away any excess water.

2   While the lentils cook, heat up the tamari or water in a saucepan or frying pan. Cook the onion and garlic until golden and the onion starts to soften. Remove from the heat and place in a mixing bowl. Add the tomato purée, smoked paprika, ground cumin, lime zest and juice, chilli flakes, if using, and seasoning to taste. Combine everything together, then add the cooked lentils and mix together well. Taste and adjust the seasoning as needed.

3   To make the guacamole, scoop the soft avocado flesh into a blender or food processor, followed by the rest of the ingredients. Blend until well combined, but leave some chunks if preferred. Taste and adjust the seasoning if necessary.

4   Serve the lentils topped with a dollop of guacamole in tortilla wraps or taco shells or use iceberg lettuce leaves for a low-carb option. Garnish with a few coriander leaves. Any leftovers can be stored in an airtight container in the fridge for three or four days, but guacamole is best eaten on the day it's made.

Thai-Spiced Veggie Burgers with a Spicy Peanut Sauce

MAKES 6–8 | BURGERS PER SERVING: 226 CALORIES | 10.3G PROTEIN | 23G CARBS | 11.3G FAT

1 large or 2 medium
sweet potatoes

3 garlic cloves, minced

8g fresh coriander,
finely chopped

6 tbsp hulled hemp seeds

2 tsp finely chopped or grated
fresh ginger

70g gluten-free rolled oats

1 x 400g tin of red kidney
beans, drained and rinsed

2 tbsp milled flaxseeds

4 tbsp cold water

juice of ½ lime

1 tbsp tamari

½ tbsp coconut oil, melted,
plus extra to grease

1 tsp smoked paprika

sea salt and freshly ground
black pepper

6–8 Portobello mushrooms,
to serve

iceberg lettuce leaves, to serve

**FOR THE SPICY PEANUT
SAUCE:**

95g smooth peanut butter
(look for an organic brand
free from added sugar and
palm oil)

1 garlic clove, peeled

juice of 1 lime

2 tbsp tamari

1 tsp finely chopped or grated
fresh ginger

5–6 drops of liquid stevia or
1 tsp honey (optional)

pinch of dried chilli flakes

sea salt and freshly ground
black pepper

dash of almond milk, to blend

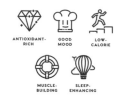

ANTIOXIDANT-RICH   GOOD MOOD   LOW-CALORIE

MUSCLE-BUILDING   SLEEP-ENHANCING

I adore Thai food and the wonderful array of herbs and spices used in traditional cooking. For this recipe I have combined some of my favourite flavours with sweet potato, kidney beans and an irresistible spicy peanut sauce.

1   Preheat the oven to 190°C. Lightly grease two baking trays with coconut oil or line with non-stick baking paper.
2   Peel the sweet potato and use a regular box grater to grate it into a large mixing bowl. Add the garlic, coriander, hemp seeds and ginger and mix together well.
3   Place the oats in a blender or food processor and blend on high for 1–2 minutes, until a coarse flour forms. Add the oat flour to the bowl with the sweet potato mixture.
4   Add the kidney beans to the blender or food processor and process until they become a coarse, chunky paste. Add them to the mixing bowl with the sweet potato and oat flour and mix well.
5   Mix together the flaxseeds and water in a small bowl to make a flax 'egg' and let it sit for 5 minutes to thicken up, then add it to the kidney bean, oat and vegetable mixture and mix well. Stir in the lime juice, tamari, melted coconut oil, smoked paprika and salt and pepper to taste.
6   Use the palms of your hands to shape the mixture into 6–8 burger patties, pressing them together to ensure they hold together well. Place each one onto one of the prepared baking trays and bake in the oven for 15–20 minutes. Flip over each burger and continue to bake for another 10–15 minutes, until golden.
7   As the burgers bake, place the Portobello mushrooms on the other prepared baking tray and roast them in the oven along with the burgers for 20–25 minutes.
8   Make the peanut sauce by adding all the sauce ingredients to a blender or food processor and blending until smooth and creamy. Taste and adjust the seasoning if necessary.
9   Serve the burgers sitting on top of the roast mushrooms or in an iceberg lettuce wrap and drizzle with peanut sauce. Store any leftovers in an airtight container in the fridge for three or four days.

Spicy Cauliflower and Corn Cakes

MAKES 6 CAKES | PER CAKE: 88 CALORIES | 3G PROTEIN | 17.2G CARBS | 1.8G FAT

coconut oil, to grease

½ head of cauliflower, chopped into florets

2 tbsp low-sodium tamari or water

1 small red onion, finely chopped

1 garlic clove, crushed

1 tsp finely chopped or grated fresh ginger

1 tbsp fresh lemon juice

1 tbsp cumin seeds

½ tsp ground turmeric

pinch of cayenne pepper

sea salt and freshly ground black pepper

240g sweetcorn

4 tbsp brown rice flour, buckwheat flour or gluten-free all-purpose flour

ANTIOXIDANT-RICH   LOW-CALORIE

This recipe came about when I didn't have much more than a tin of sweetcorn in the cupboard and a cauliflower in the fridge, but it turned out to be a really tasty, low-calorie meal. As always, I've used plenty of herbs and spices rather than oil to create flavour, and I love the combination of garlic, ginger and cumin seeds.

1   Preheat the oven to 190°C. Line a baking tray with non-stick baking paper or lightly grease with coconut oil.

2   Place the cauliflower in a medium saucepan and cover with water. Bring to the boil for 2–3 minutes, then lower the temperature and simmer for 5–6 minutes, until soft. Drain well.

3   Heat the tamari or water in a frying pan and add the onion, garlic and ginger. Cook for 4–5 minutes, until the onion softens. Lower the temperature to medium-low and add the lemon juice, cumin seeds, turmeric, cayenne pepper and salt and pepper. Stir gently for 2–3 minutes, then remove from the heat.

4   Place the cauliflower and sweetcorn in a medium-sized mixing bowl, then add the warm onion, ginger, garlic and spice mixture. Use a potato masher to mash all the ingredients together well, then stir in the flour to thicken it up and form a dough. Add a little more flour if it's too wet or sticky.

5   Divide the dough into 6 patties, using the palms of your hands to flatten and shape them, then place them on the prepared baking tray.

6   Bake in the oven for 20–25 minutes, until golden brown. Serve warm with a big green salad. Any leftovers can be stored in an airtight container in the fridge for three or four days.

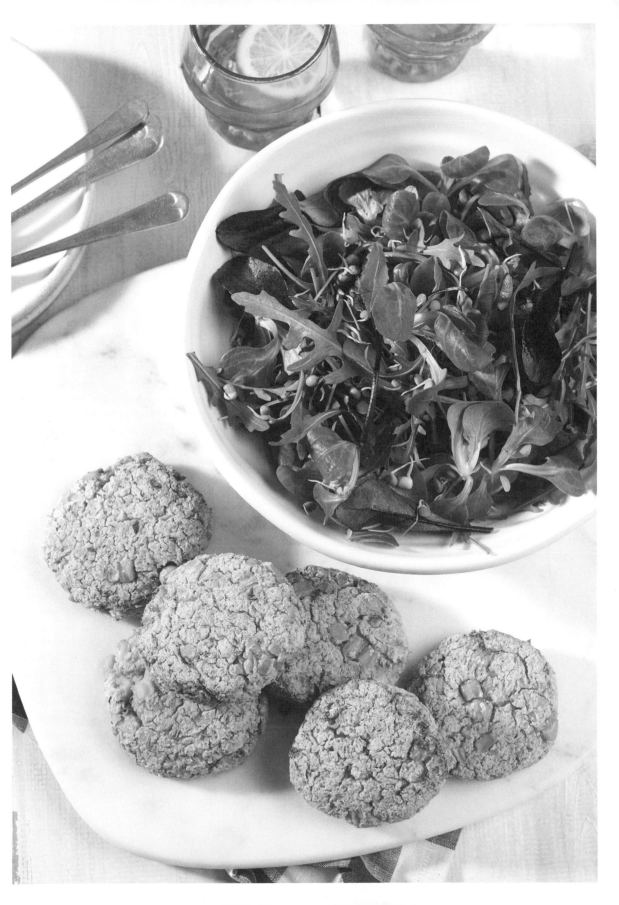

Smoky Falafel Burgers

MAKES 6–8 | PER BURGER: 97 CALORIES | 5.6G PROTEIN | 15.8G CARBS | 1.4G FAT

coconut oil, to grease

1 x 400g tin of cooked chickpeas, drained and rinsed

1 medium carrot, roughly chopped

½ red onion, roughly chopped

2 garlic cloves, peeled

1 tsp minced fresh ginger

2 tbsp nutritional yeast (optional)

2 tsp smoked paprika

1 tsp ground cumin

1 tsp ground coriander or a small handful of fresh coriander

pinch of cayenne pepper or dried chilli flakes (optional)

sea salt and freshly ground black pepper

4 tbsp chickpea flour (gram flour)

2–3 tbsp unsweetened almond milk or any other plant milk

TO SERVE:

hummus (page 227 or page 228)

gluten-free pitta bread, iceberg lettuce or red cabbage leaves

These healthy falafel-style burgers are delicious with a dollop of sun-dried tomato hummus (see the recipe on page 227) in a pitta bread or in an iceberg lettuce or red cabbage wrap for a lower-carb version. The smoked paprika and metabolism-boosting cayenne pepper deliver a double dose of antioxidants, while the chickpeas, grated carrot and chickpea flour add to this meal's protein, fibre and slow-energy release. I use chickpea flour, but rice flour, buckwheat flour, oat flour and gluten-free all-purpose flour also work well.

1 Preheat the oven to 200°C. Line a baking tray with non-stick baking paper or lightly grease with coconut oil.

2 Place the chickpeas in a food processor with the carrot, onion, garlic and ginger. Process until a coarsely ground mixture is formed. Transfer to a bowl and add the nutritional yeast, if using, spices and seasoning. Mix well. Add the flour and almond milk, stirring until the mixture thickens up. Taste and adjust the seasoning as needed.

3 Use the palms of your hands to roll the mixture into 6–8 burger patties and place on the baking tray. Bake in the oven for 18–20 minutes, until they begin to crisp up and turn golden brown on the outside. Remove from the oven and allow them to cool.

4 Serve with a dollop of hummus in a gluten-free pitta bread or an iceberg lettuce or red cabbage shell.

5 Any leftovers can be stored in an airtight container in the fridge for three or four days.

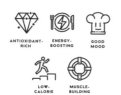

ANTIOXIDANT-RICH   ENERGY-BOOSTING   GOOD MOOD

LOW-CALORIE   MUSCLE-BUILDING

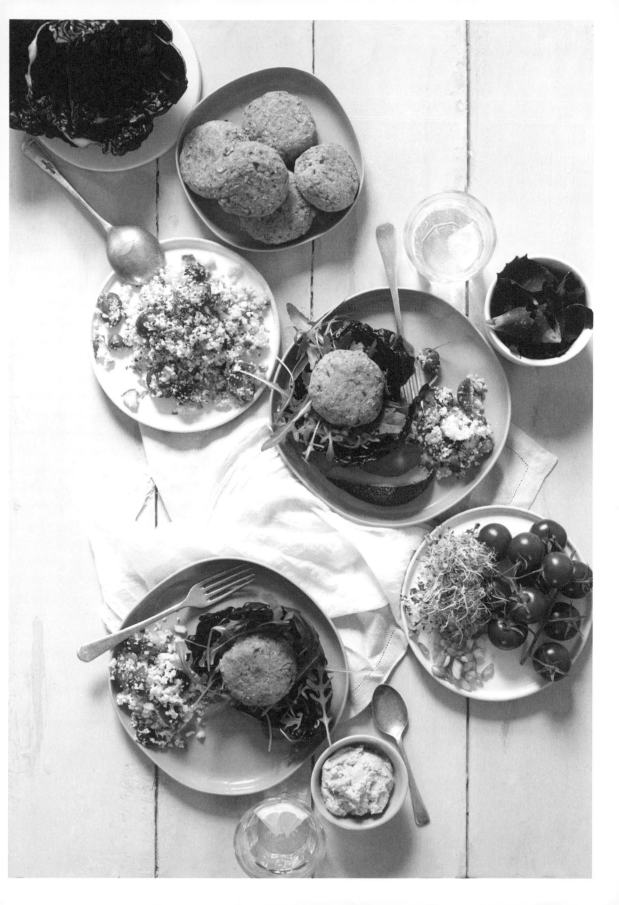

Avocado, Lemon and Basil
Pesto Courgetti

SERVES 2 | PER SERVING: 255 CALORIES | 9.4G PROTEIN | 19.9G CARBS | 17.7G FAT

2 medium-large courgettes

1 ripe avocado, halved
and pitted

1 large garlic clove, peeled

2 large handfuls of fresh basil

1 handful of fresh mint leaves

2 tbsp nutritional yeast

2 tbsp fresh lemon juice

2 tbsp tamari

1 tsp smoked paprika

pinch of dried chilli flakes
(optional)

sea salt and freshly ground
black pepper

1 tbsp hulled hemp seeds

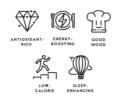

ANTIOXIDANT-RICH   ENERGY-BOOSTING   GOOD MOOD

LOW-CALORIE   SLEEP-ENHANCING

Quick, healthy, fresh and zesty, this is one of my favourite simple
and light yet filling meals. During the week I try to eat as cleanly as
possible to really maximise the benefits of my workouts, so I always
stock up on courgettes for quick courgetti lunches and dinners. The
heart-healthy fats, essential minerals and antioxidant vitamins found
in the avocado help to build a smooth and soft complexion, while the
protein in the hemp seeds goes towards muscle recovery and repair.

1   Cut the ends off the courgettes and use a spiraliser or vegetable
    peeler to process them into noodles or ribbons. Place them in a
    large mixing bowl and set aside.
2   Place all the remaining ingredients apart from the hemp seeds into
    a blender or food processor and blitz until smooth and creamy.
    Pour the pesto into the bowl with the courgetti and mix together
    well, until the noodles are well coated.
3   Divide between two bowls and top with the hulled hemp seeds.
    Any leftovers can be stored in an airtight container in the fridge
    for up to three days.

Chickpea and Sesame Cakes with Spicy Mango Salsa

SERVES 2 | PER SERVING: 508 CALORIES | 20G PROTEIN | 82.7G CARBS | 14.2G FAT

1 tbsp ground flaxseeds

2 tbsp cold water

1 x 400g tin of chickpeas, drained and rinsed

25g chickpea flour, rice flour, buckwheat flour or gluten-free all-purpose flour

1 red onion, finely sliced

1 garlic clove, minced

2 tbsp sesame seeds

1 tbsp whole chia seeds

1 tbsp pumpkin seeds

1 tsp ground cumin

1 tsp smoked paprika

pinch of cayenne pepper (optional)

sea salt and freshly ground black pepper

1 tsp coconut oil

FOR THE SPICY MANGO SALSA:

1 mango, peeled, cored and cut into cubes

8 cherry tomatoes, quartered

½ red onion, finely chopped

1 jalapeño, deseeded and finely chopped

2 handfuls of fresh coriander, chopped

1 handful of fresh mint leaves, chopped

2 tbsp fresh lime juice

sea salt and freshly ground black pepper

Chunky chickpeas add a hearty bite to these wholesome savoury cakes and I love the juicy, fresh flavours of the spicy mango salsa. Pop a few on top of a big green salad for a healthy and satisfying meal.

1 In a small bowl, mix together the flaxseeds and water. Set aside for 5 minutes to set into a flax 'egg'.

2 Place the flax 'egg' and all the remaining ingredients except the coconut oil into a food processor. Process until a sticky and slightly chunky mixture forms that will stick together when pressed between your fingers. Use the palms of your hands to form the mixture into 4 patties, making them as smooth and even as possible, pressing them firmly together to ensure they won't break apart.

3 In a medium frying pan set over a medium-high heat, heat up the coconut oil and fry the patties for 4–5 minutes, until they're golden brown on both sides. Place them on a piece of kitchen paper when cooked to soak up any excess oil.

4 To make the spicy mango salsa, simply toss all the ingredients together in a mixing bowl and adjust the seasoning as needed.

5 Serve the chickpea and sesame cakes warm with the mango salsa and a big green salad. They also work well cold as a packed lunch option. Any leftovers can be stored in an airtight container in the fridge for up to three days.

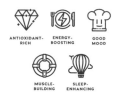

ANTIOXIDANT-RICH   ENERGY-BOOSTING   GOOD MOOD   MUSCLE-BUILDING   SLEEP-ENHANCING

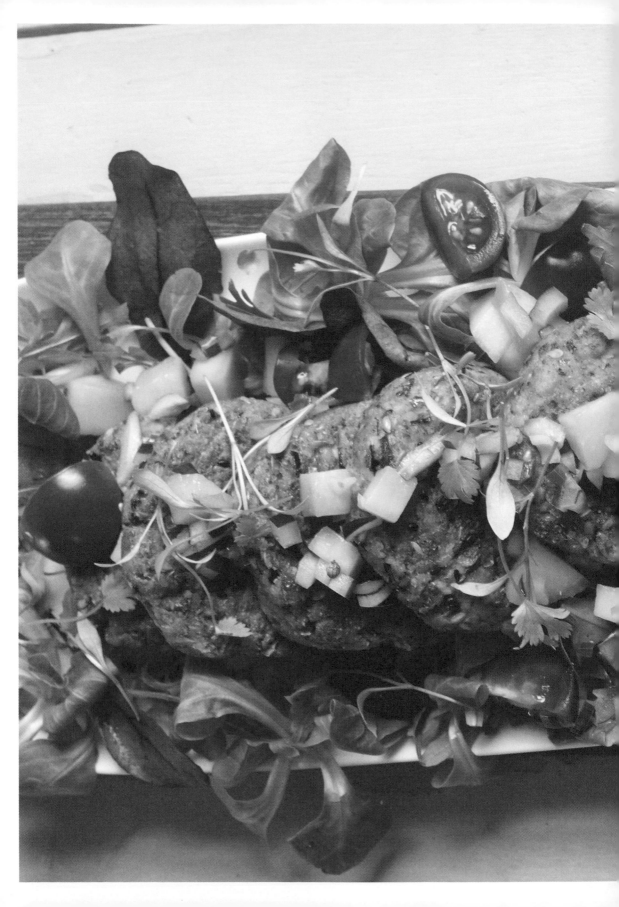

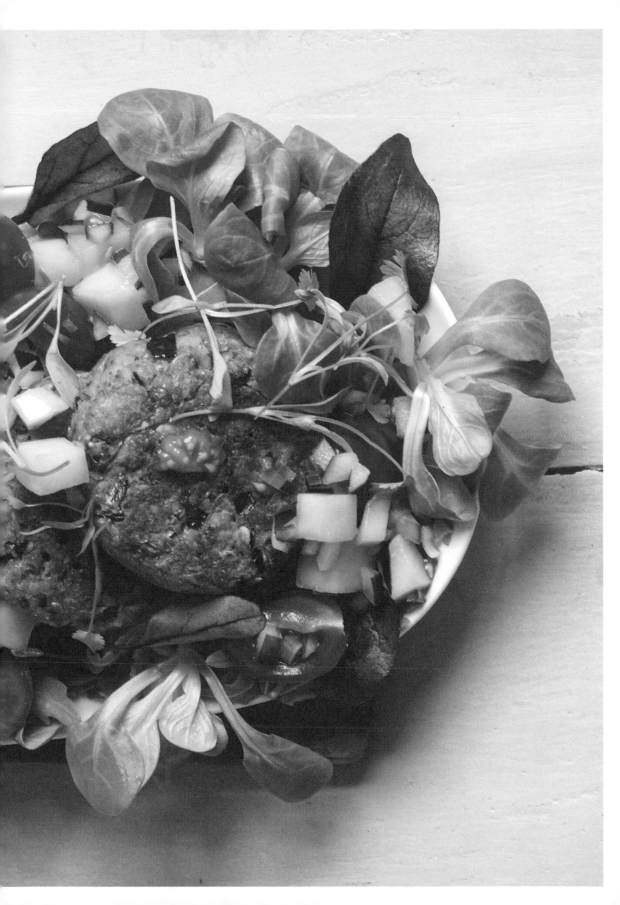

Black Bean and Sweet Potato Chilli

SERVES 2 | PER SERVING: 333 CALORIES | 14.4G PROTEIN | 70G CARBS | 1G FAT

coconut oil, to grease

2 medium-large
sweet potatoes

2 tbsp low-sodium tamari
or water

1 red onion, finely sliced

1 red pepper, chopped

1 garlic clove, minced

1 x 400g tin of black beans,
drained and rinsed

160g tomato passata

1 tsp Cajun spices

1 tsp ground coriander

1 tsp smoked paprika

½ tsp ground cumin

pinch of cayenne pepper

sea salt and freshly ground
black pepper

1 handful of baby spinach

chopped fresh parsley,
to garnish

I adore the combination of flavours in this chilli, which include Cajun spices, coriander, cumin, smoked paprika and a pinch of cayenne pepper to give it a little bit of bite. Black beans are a super source of protein, with 10.6g per serving. I love this chilli served hot over a baked sweet potato for a hearty, healthy and filling good mood meal packed with protein, complex carbs and fibre.

1   Preheat the oven to 200°C. Lightly grease a baking tray with coconut oil or line with non-stick baking paper.
2   Place the sweet potatoes on the baking tray and bake in the oven for 35–40 minutes, until they're soft and easy to slice.
3   Meanwhile, heat the tamari or water in a saucepan set over a medium heat and cook the onion, pepper and garlic for 3–4 minutes, until the vegetables soften. Stir in the black beans, tomato passata, spices and seasoning and gently simmer the chilli for another 5 minutes, until heated through. Remove from the heat and mix in the spinach leaves, allowing them to wilt.
4   When the sweet potatoes are baked, allow them to cool for 5–10 minutes before slicing them down the middle lengthways, but don't cut them all the way through. Open them out a bit, then spoon on the chilli and garnish with plenty of chopped fresh parsley.

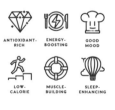

ANTIOXIDANT-RICH   ENERGY-BOOSTING   GOOD MOOD   LOW-CALORIE   MUSCLE-BUILDING   SLEEP-ENHANCING

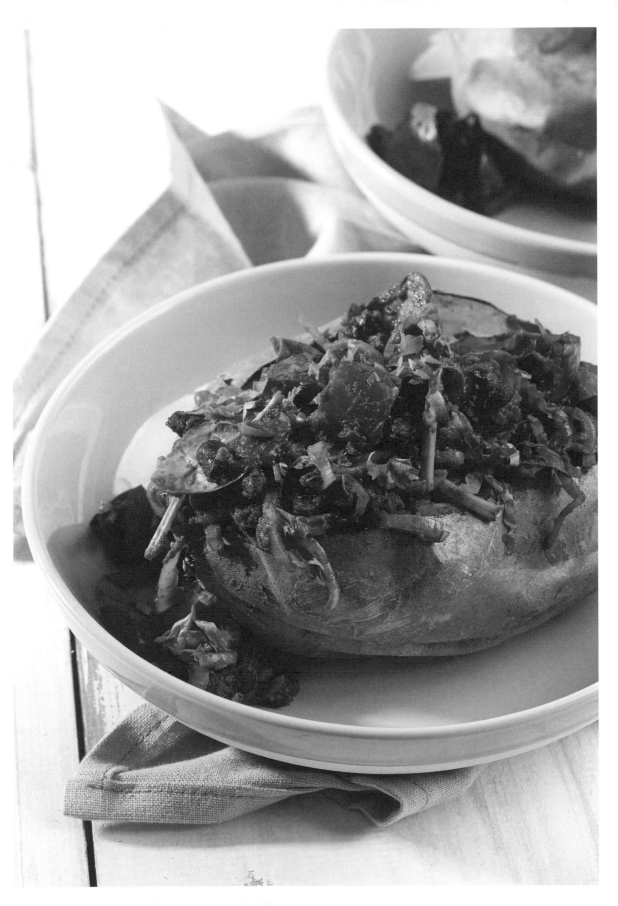

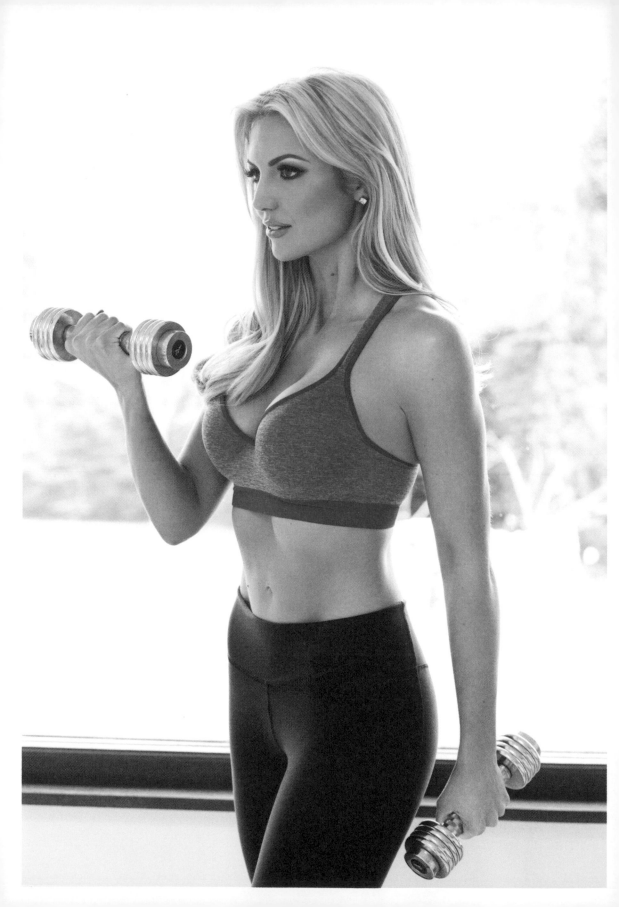

Chilli san Carne

SERVES 4–6 | PER SERVING: 221 CALORIES | 10.7G PROTEIN | 41G CARBS | 1.3G FAT

1 medium butternut squash

2 tbsp low-sodium tamari or water

1 red onion, finely chopped

2 garlic cloves, minced

1 x 400g tin of red kidney beans, drained and rinsed

1 x 400g tin of adzuki or black-eyed beans, drained and rinsed

800g tomato passata

250ml low-fat coconut milk or unsweetened almond milk

2 tbsp fresh lemon juice

1 tbsp ground cumin

2–3 tsp smoked paprika

½ tsp dried chilli flakes

sea salt and freshly ground black pepper

65g fresh kale, tough stems removed

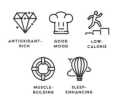

ANTIOXIDANT-RICH   GOOD MOOD   LOW-CALORIE   MUSCLE-BUILDING   SLEEP-ENHANCING

The array of spices in this nourishing meal incorporates lots of flavour, and I add kale for its incredible range of antioxidants and minerals. This is a great dish to make in a big batch at the beginning of the week and it works especially well to warm you up on chilly winter nights.

1   Preheat the oven to 200°C.

2   Place the whole butternut squash on a baking tray. Roast for 30–35 minutes, until its skin turns golden brown. Remove from the heat and set aside to cool for 10 minutes. When it has cooled enough to handle, peel the skin off the squash, cut it in half and scoop out the seeds and pulp in the middle, then cut the flesh into bite-sized chunks.

3   In a large saucepan set over a medium heat, heat up the tamari or water and cook the onion and garlic for 4–5 minutes, until the onion starts to soften. Add the chopped butternut squash and continue to sauté for another 2–3 minutes. Add the beans, tomato passata, coconut milk, lemon juice, ground cumin, smoked paprika, chilli flakes and seasoning. Bring to the boil for 2–3 minutes, then lower the heat, partly cover with a lid and simmer for about 15 minutes, until the mixture has thickened and heated through. Stir regularly to prevent it from burning and add extra coconut milk or water if you prefer a runnier texture. Remove from the heat and stir in the kale, allowing the leaves to wilt.

4   Divide into serving bowls and serve hot. Any leftovers can be stored in an airtight container in the fridge for three or four days.

Spicy Tomato, Chickpea and Courgetti Bolognese

SERVES 2 | PER SERVING: 334 CALORIES | 16.4G PROTEIN | 48G CARBS | 11G FAT

2 medium courgettes

2 tbsp fresh lemon juice

Himalayan pink rock salt and freshly ground black pepper

2 tbsp low-sodium tamari or water

1 red onion, finely sliced

2 garlic cloves, minced

180g cooked or tinned chickpeas, drained and rinsed

125ml tomato passata

2 tbsp nutritional yeast

1 tsp coriander seeds

1 tsp ground cumin

1 tsp smoked paprika, plus extra to garnish

pinch of cayenne pepper

2 handfuls of fresh basil leaves

½ ripe avocado, pitted, peeled and cut into cubes

dash of tamari

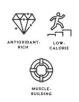

ANTIOXIDANT-RICH   LOW-CALORIE

MUSCLE-BUILDING

Light, summery, healthy and fresh with a hint of chilli, this dish is so easy to whip up for a light lunch or dinner. It's ideal for those trying to tone up and lose body fat as chickpeas are a perfect food for anyone watching their weight. They're low in calories and filled with protein and fibre to help repair torn muscle fibres and stabilise blood sugar levels. I add cubes of avocado for an extra dose of heart-healthy fats and minerals, including potassium and magnesium.

1   Use a spiraliser or vegetable peeler to create the courgetti noodles. Add the lemon juice and a pinch of salt, toss it all together and set aside.

2   In a saucepan set over a medium heat, heat up the tamari or water and cook the onion and garlic for 3–4 minutes, until the onion softens. Add the chickpeas and stir for 1 minute, then add the tomato passata, nutritional yeast, coriander seeds, ground cumin, smoked paprika, cayenne pepper and seasoning. Allow it to simmer gently for about 10 minutes, stirring frequently. Remove the saucepan from the heat and add the basil, stirring to allow it to gently wilt.

3   Serve the Bolognese over the courgetti, topped with avocado cubes, a drizzle of tamari and a sprinkle of smoked paprika. Leftovers will keep in a covered container in the fridge for up to two days.

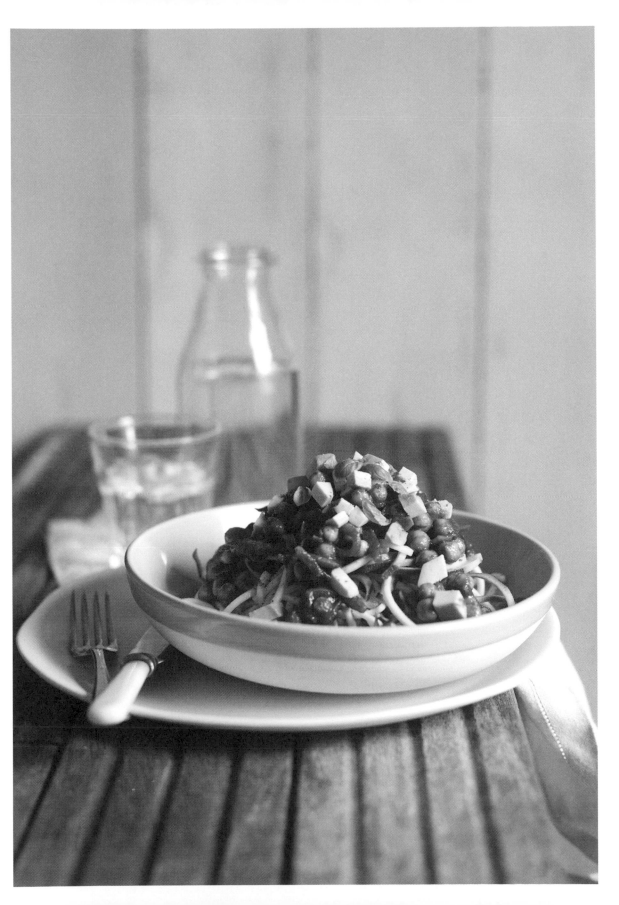

Vindaloo Vegetables with Ginger and Lime Cauliflower Rice

SERVES 4 | PER SERVING: 271 CALORIES | 16.9G PROTEIN | 52G CARBS | 1.5G FAT

2 tbsp low-sodium tamari or water

2 carrots, thinly sliced

1 medium red onion, chopped

1 small to medium head of cauliflower, cut into small florets

2 x 400g tins of red kidney beans, drained and rinsed

170g tomato purée

185ml water

2 small courgettes, cut into 6mm-thick slices

1 green, yellow or red bell pepper, deseeded and diced

sea salt and freshly ground black pepper

135g frozen peas, thawed

FOR THE SPICE PASTE:

3 garlic cloves, peeled

1 tbsp tamari

1 tbsp chopped fresh ginger

1½ tsp ground coriander

1¼ tsp ground cumin

½ tsp ground turmeric

¼ tsp cardamom

pinch of dried chilli flakes

125ml cold water

FOR THE GINGER AND LIME CAULIFLOWER RICE:

1 large cauliflower, roughly chopped

zest and juice of 1 lime

2 tbsp chopped fresh coriander, plus extra to garnish

1 tbsp grated fresh ginger

ANTIOXIDANT-RICH   LOW-CALORIE

MUSCLE-BUILDING

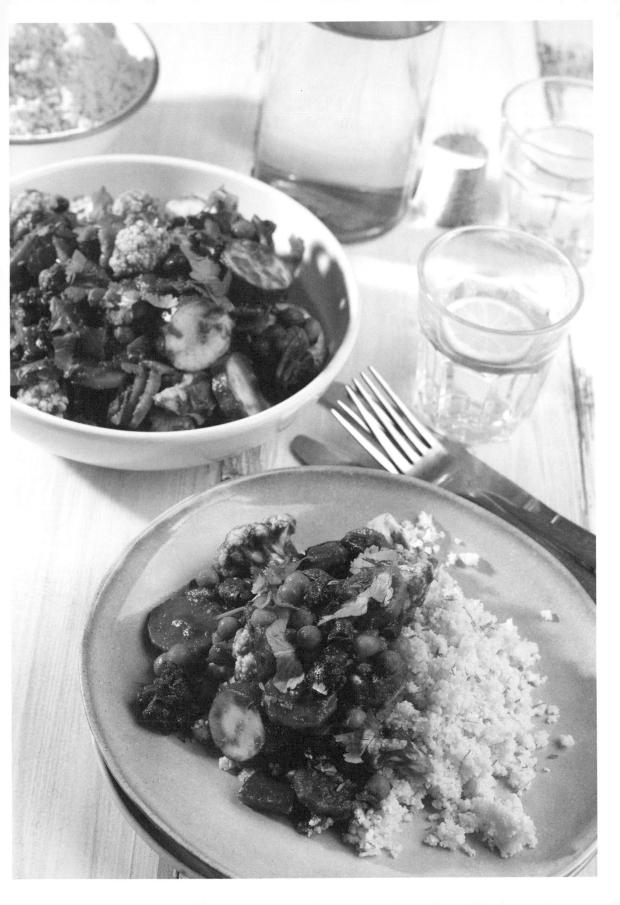

This protein-packed, low-carb and oil-free dish is bursting with flavour from the array of herbs and spices used, all of which have health-promoting properties. This filling and fibre-rich dish is ideal for making in a big batch and enjoying over two or three days. It works well as a cold packed lunch or it can be gently reheated in the oven for an evening meal.

1   To make the spice paste, place the garlic, tamari, ginger, coriander, cumin, turmeric, cardamom, chilli flakes and water in a blender or food processor. Combine until a smooth paste forms and set aside.

2   In a large saucepan set over a medium-high heat, heat up the tamari or water. Add the chopped carrots and onion and cook for 4–5 minutes, until the vegetables have softened, stirring frequently to prevent them from burning. Add more water if necessary. Add the spice paste and cook for about 2 minutes, stirring continuously. Add the cauliflower and kidney beans, then cover the saucepan and lower the heat.

3   Put the tomato purée and water into the blender and blitz until smooth, then pour this into the vegetables. Cover with a lid and cook for 5 minutes, then add the courgettes and bell pepper. Season with a pinch of sea salt and pepper, cover the saucepan again and continue cooking for 5–10 minutes more, until the vegetables are tender and well combined with the spices. Add the thawed peas and allow them to heat up for 2–3 minutes.

4   To make the cauliflower rice, put the roughly chopped cauliflower into a blender or food processor and process for 2–3 minutes, until it forms a rice-like consistency. Heat 1–2 tablespoons of water in a large frying pan, then add the lime zest, coriander and ginger. Stir for 30 seconds, then add the cauliflower rice, 3 more tablespoons of water and the lime juice. Cook for 5 minutes, until fully cooked through.

5   Divide the cauliflower rice between four plates and serve the vindaloo vegetables on the side, garnished with chopped fresh coriander.

Coconut Curried Quinoa with Cheesy Roast Cauliflower

SERVES 4 | PER SERVING: 291 CALORIES | 13.3G PROTEIN | 47.3G CARBS | 7.2G FAT

2 tbsp low-sodium tamari or water

1 medium red onion, finely sliced

1 garlic clove, minced

1 tbsp curry powder

1 tsp grated or finely chopped fresh ginger or ground ginger

1 tsp ground turmeric

400ml low-fat coconut milk

125ml water

170g quinoa, rinsed well under cold water

3 tbsp raisins (optional)

sea salt and freshly ground black pepper

80g fresh rocket leaves

FOR THE CHEESY ROAST CAULIFLOWER:

2 heaped tbsp nutritional yeast

2 tbsp fresh lemon juice

2 tsp coconut oil, melted, plus extra for greasing

1 tsp smoked paprika

pinch of cayenne pepper (optional)

2 small or 1 medium head of cauliflower, cut into bite-sized florets

This filling dish is brilliant to make in a bigger batch and eat over a couple of days, as it keeps well in the fridge and even tastes great cold. The cheesy roast cauliflower makes a deliciously satisfying topping for the quinoa and the spices used create a rich flavour.

1   To cook the cheesy cauliflower, preheat the oven to 190°C. Lightly grease a large baking tray with coconut oil or line with non-stick baking paper.

2   In a large mixing bowl, stir together the nutritional yeast, lemon juice, melted coconut oil, smoked paprika, cayenne pepper, if using, and some salt and pepper. Add the cauliflower pieces and toss together well, ensuring that each piece is covered in the mixture.

3   Spread the cauliflower out on the tray and roast in the oven for 25–30 minutes, until golden brown and crisp, turning them over halfway through.

4   Meanwhile, heat the tamari or water in a large saucepan, then add the onion and garlic. Cook for 4–5 minutes, until the onion begins to soften. Add the curry powder, ginger and turmeric and stir for about 30 seconds, until fragrant. Pour in the coconut milk, water, quinoa and raisins, if using. Bring to the boil for 2–3 minutes, then cover partly with a lid and reduce the heat to a simmer.

5   Simmer for 15 minutes, until the quinoa seeds have opened out, then remove the saucepan from the heat and let it sit for 5 minutes so that the quinoa can absorb any remaining liquid. Use a fork to fluff up the quinoa, then season to taste and stir in the rocket leaves.

6   To serve, divide the quinoa between four bowls and top with the roasted cauliflower. Any leftovers can be stored in an airtight container in the fridge for three or four days.

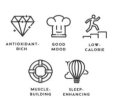

ANTIOXIDANT-RICH   GOOD MOOD   LOW-CALORIE

MUSCLE-BUILDING   SLEEP-ENHANCING

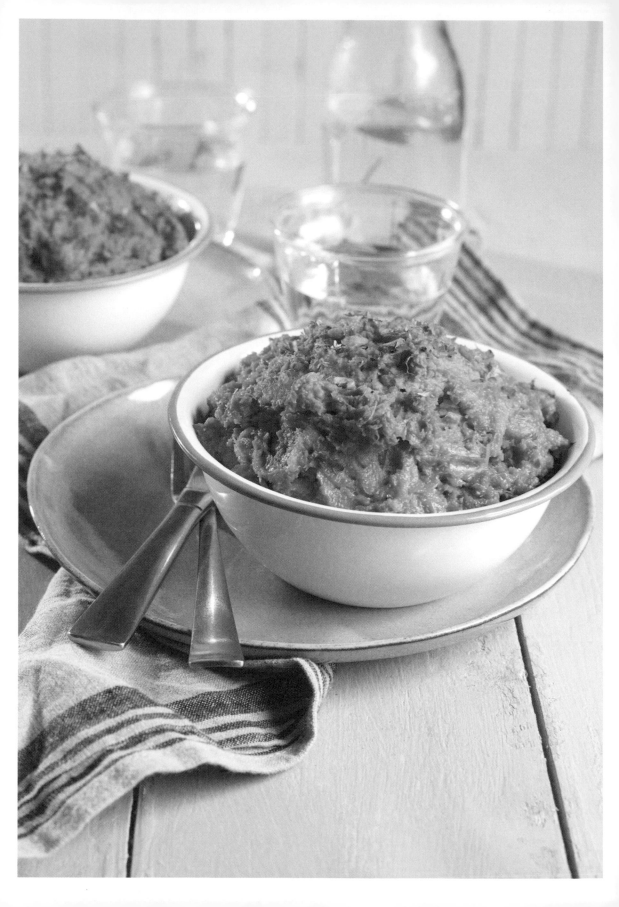

Lentil and Cheesy Cumin Sweet Potato Pies

SERVES 2 | PER SERVING: 481 CALORIES | 27.8G PROTEIN | 93.6G CARBS | 2.4G FAT

FOR THE CHEESY CUMIN SWEET POTATO CRUST:

2 medium sweet potatoes, peeled and cut into chunks

2 heaped tbsp nutritional yeast

1–2 tsp ground cumin

1 tsp smoked paprika

sea salt and freshly ground black pepper

chopped fresh parsley, to garnish

FOR THE LENTIL FILLING:

2 tbsp low-sodium tamari or water

2 medium red onions, diced

2 garlic cloves, minced

4 medium carrots, diced

1½ x 400g tins of chopped tomatoes

1½ x 400g tins of Puy lentils, drained and rinsed

250ml low-sodium vegetable stock

2 tbsp tomato purée

2 tsp ground cumin

2 tsp ground coriander

1 tsp dried oregano

pinch of dried chilli flakes

These steaming hot and hearty pies filled with a lentil and tomato stew and topped with cheesy cumin mash make a wonderfully warming and satisfying meal. Good mood food at its best.

1   Preheat the oven to 200°C.

2   Place the sweet potatoes in a medium saucepan set over a medium-high heat. Cover with water and bring to the boil, then reduce to a simmer and cook for 8–10 minutes, until the potatoes are tender enough to slice with a knife. Drain away the water and place them back in the saucepan with the nutritional yeast, ground cumin, smoked paprika and seasoning and mash well, until fluffy.

3   Heat the tamari or water in a large saucepan set over a medium-high heat and cook the onions and garlic for 3–4 minutes, until soft and translucent. Add the carrots and continue to cook until the vegetables have softened, stirring often. Add the chopped tomatoes, lentils, vegetable stock, tomato purée, spices and some salt and pepper and bring the mixture to the boil for 2–3 minutes. Reduce the heat to a simmer, cover the saucepan partly with a lid and cook for another 12–15 minutes, until the mixture has reduced and thickened.

4   Divide the lentil and vegetable mixture between two ovenproof serving bowls and top with the mashed sweet potatoes. Bake in the oven for 15–20 minutes, until the tops are golden and crispy. Allow to cool for 5 minutes and serve hot, garnished with fresh parsley. Any leftovers can be stored in an airtight container in the fridge for three or four days.

ANTIOXIDANT-RICH   GOOD MOOD

MUSCLE-BUILDING   SLEEP-ENHANCING

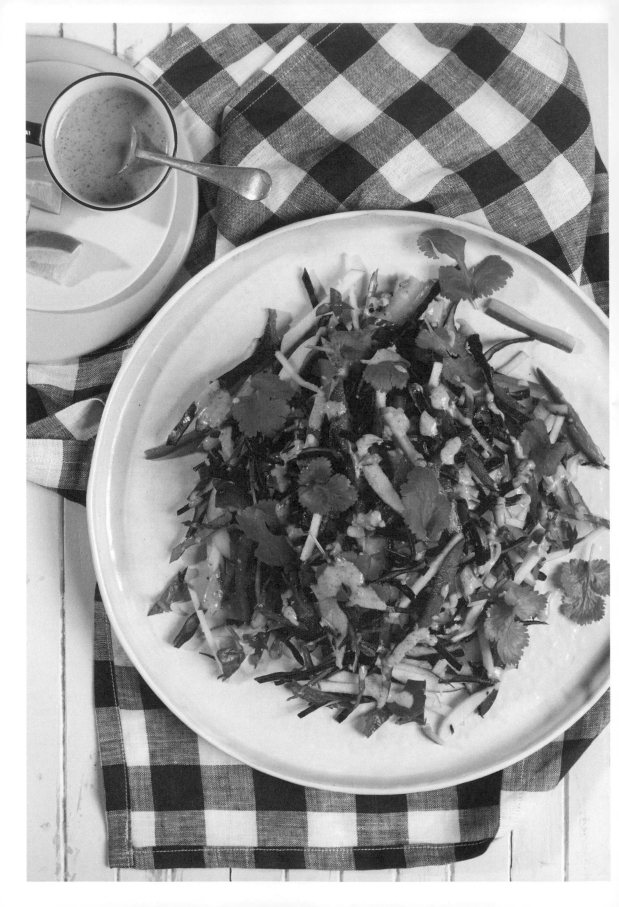

Vegetable Pad Thai with a Spicy Almond Sauce

SERVES 2 | PER SERVING: 388 CALORIES | 12G PROTEIN | 33.9G CARBS | 26.4G FAT

70g red cabbage, shredded or finely chopped

60g baby spinach, shredded or finely chopped

8g fresh coriander leaves

1–2 tbsp fresh lime juice

sea salt and freshly ground black pepper

2 garlic cloves, minced

4 tbsp tamari

1 tbsp red wine vinegar

2 tsp minced or finely chopped fresh ginger

1 tsp coconut oil, melted

pinch of dried chilli flakes (optional)

1 green apple, thinly sliced

1 red bell pepper, cored and thinly sliced

½ red onion, finely sliced

½ medium cucumber, finely sliced

lime wedges, to serve

FOR THE SPICY ALMOND SAUCE:

85g raw unsalted almond butter (use tahini or sunflower seed butter for a nut-free version)

2 garlic cloves, minced

3–4 tbsp water, to blend

2 tbsp fresh lemon juice

1 tbsp grated fresh ginger

1 tbsp tamari

1 tbsp pure maple syrup or honey or 5–6 drops of liquid stevia (optional)

pinch of dried chilli flakes (optional)

sea salt and freshly ground black pepper

I love the array of flavours in this recipe, based on a range of different veggies, herbs and spices. Drizzle with a generous amount of the spicy almond sauce for a healthy and satisfying meal.

1   Place the cabbage, spinach, coriander and lime juice in a large mixing bowl. Season and set aside.
2   Whisk together the garlic, tamari, vinegar, ginger, melted coconut oil and the chilli flakes, if using, in a smaller bowl and set aside.
3   Add the apple, pepper, onion and cucumber to the cabbage, then top with the tamari dressing and mix everything together well.
4   Make the spicy almond sauce by placing all the ingredients in a blender or food processor and blitzing until smooth and creamy, using more water if necessary. Taste and adjust the seasoning as needed.
5   Serve the pad Thai drizzled with spicy almond sauce and lime wedges on the side. Any leftovers can be stored in an airtight container in the fridge for three or four days.

Roast Aubergine Curry with Basil and Toasted Cashews

SERVES 2 | PER SERVING: 329 CALORIES | 11.4G PROTEIN | 52.5G CARBS | 11.8G FAT

coconut oil, to grease

1 aubergine, cut into chunks

1 medium-large or 2 small sweet potatoes, peeled and cut into chunks

4 tbsp unsalted raw cashews

2 tbsp low-sodium tamari or water

1 red onion, finely chopped

1 garlic clove, minced

1 tsp chopped fresh ginger

2 tsp curry powder

500g tomato passata

500ml Koko coconut milk

1 tsp ground turmeric

1 tsp ground coriander

pinch of dried chilli flakes

sea salt and freshly ground black pepper

1 large handful of fresh basil, torn

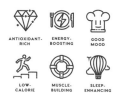

ANTIOXIDANT-RICH   ENERGY-BOOSTING   GOOD MOOD

LOW-CALORIE   MUSCLE-BUILDING   SLEEP-ENHANCING

One of my favourite ways to eat aubergine, this is a warming and satisfying curry featuring baked sweet potato and an array of fragrant spices. Toasted cashews add a satisfying crunch, and it's filing enough to eat by itself or with a side of brown rice.

1   Preheat the oven to 190°C. Lightly grease a large baking tray with coconut oil.

2   Spread out the aubergine and sweet potato on the baking tray. Roast them in the oven for 25–30 minutes, until the potato turns golden brown and crisp. Set aside.

3   While the vegetables roast, spread the cashews out on a small baking tray and toast in the oven for 10 minutes, until golden. Set aside.

4   In a large saucepan set over a medium heat, heat up the tamari or water and add the onion, garlic and ginger. Cook for 3–4 minutes, until the onion is beginning to soften, then add the curry powder and stir for another 1–2 minutes. Add the roast aubergine and sweet potato chunks and stir for 1 minute, then add the tomato passata and coconut milk.

5   Mix well to combine all the ingredients and bring to the boil for 1–2 minutes. Reduce the temperature to a simmer and stir in the turmeric, coriander, chilli flakes and seasoning. Partly cover the saucepan with a lid and simmer for another 10–12 minutes, until heated through. Remove from the heat and stir in the basil leaves, allowing them to gently wilt.

6   Serve hot, topped with toasted cashews. Any leftovers can be stored in an airtight container in the fridge for three or four days.

Butternut Squash and Sage Risotto

SERVES 4 | PER SERVING: 288 CALORIES | 8G PROTEIN | 60G CARBS | 3.5G FAT

coconut oil, to grease

1 butternut squash

4 tbsp low-sodium tamari

2 garlic cloves, minced

sea salt and freshly ground
black pepper

200g Arborio rice

1 litre hot vegetable stock

2 tbsp nutritional yeast
(optional)

1 tbsp chopped fresh sage or
1 tsp dried sage

2 tbsp toasted pine nuts,
to serve

2 tbsp chopped fresh parsley,
to garnish

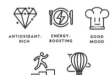

ANTIOXIDANT-
RICH   ENERGY-
BOOSTING   GOOD
MOOD

LOW-
CALORIE   SLEEP-
ENHANCING

Hearty, wholesome and seriously satisfying, risotto is a universally popular comfort meal. I've combined the natural sweetness of roast butternut squash with sage to pack in plenty of flavour and nutrients. Butternut squash is a superb source of beta-carotene for a healthy and glowing complexion.

1   Preheat the oven to 200°C. Lightly grease a baking tray with coconut oil or line with a sheet of non-stick baking paper.

2   Place the whole butternut squash on the tray and roast for 30–35 minutes, until the skin of the squash has turned golden brown. Remove it from the heat and let it cool for 10 minutes. When it's cool enough to handle, peel off the skin, cut it in half to scoop out the seeds, then cut the flesh into bite-sized cubes.

3   In a saucepan set over a medium heat, heat up 2 tablespoons of the tamari (or water) and cook the garlic until it's golden. Add the butternut squash cubes and season with a pinch of sea salt and black pepper. Continue to sauté over a medium-high heat for a few minutes more, until the squash begins to soften. Reduce to a medium heat, add the rice into the squash and stir for 1–2 minutes, until the rice begins to turn opaque.

4   Add the stock to the saucepan 125ml at a time, stirring it in. As it begins to evaporate, add the next 125ml. Keep repeating until the rice has cooked and become smooth and creamy.

5   Stir in the nutritional yeast, the remaining 2 tablespoons of tamari and the sage and season with a pinch of salt and pepper as needed. Top with toasted pine nuts and chopped parsley and serve hot. Any leftovers can be stored in an airtight container in the fridge for up to three days.

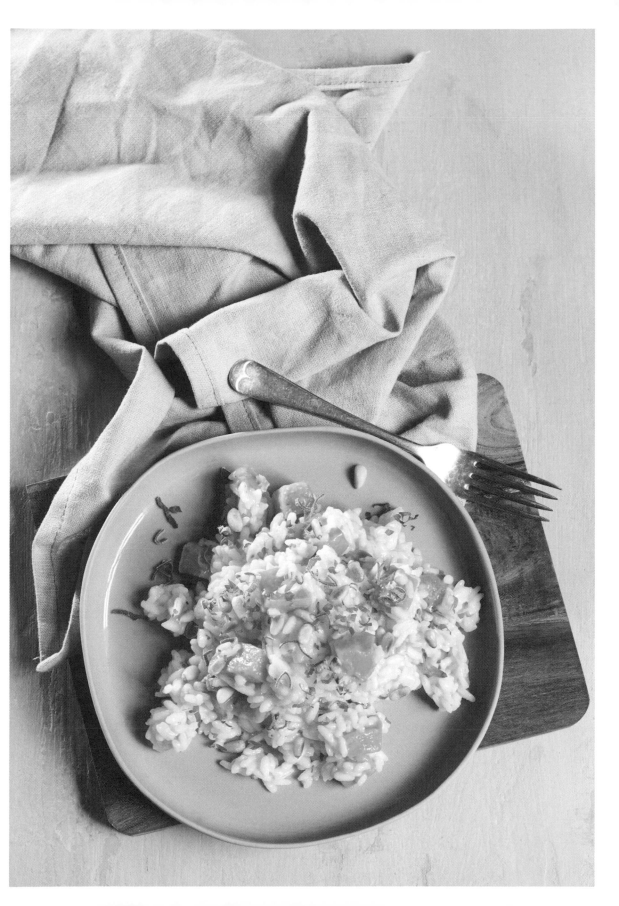

Portobello Mushroom and Sweet Potato Pie with Pine Nut Parmesan

SERVES 6–8 | PER SERVING: 465 CALORIES | 10.7G PROTEIN | 73.2G CARBS | 15G FAT

FOR THE PIE CRUST:

360g spelt flour or gluten-free all-purpose flour

6 tsp gluten-free baking powder

pinch of sea salt

4 tbsp coconut oil, at room temperature, plus extra for greasing

170ml boiling water

FOR THE SWEET POTATO TOPPING:

6 small or medium sweet potatoes, peeled and chopped into chunks

3 tbsp nutritional yeast (optional)

1 tbsp coconut oil

4 tsp smoked paprika

FOR THE MUSHROOM FILLING:

2 tbsp low-sodium tamari or water

1 red onion, finely sliced

1 garlic clove, minced

1 medium carrot, cut into bite-sized slices

200ml low-sodium vegetable stock

125ml red wine

3 tsp dried thyme

pinch of dried chilli flakes

455g Portobello mushrooms, rinsed well and sliced

3 tbsp nutritional yeast (or 2 tbsp gluten-free all-purpose flour)

sea salt and freshly ground black pepper

FOR THE PINE NUT PARMESAN:

2 tbsp pine nuts, lightly toasted

2 tbsp nutritional yeast

sea salt and freshly ground black pepper

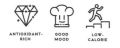

ANTIOXIDANT-RICH GOOD MOOD LOW-CALORIE

MUSCLE-BUILDING SLEEP-ENHANCING

This wholesome pie is filled with the meaty texture of Portobello mushrooms and topped with a crisp sweet potato mash. Perfect for making as a big family meal on a chilly evening.

1   To make the pie crust, lightly grease a 20cm pie dish with coconut oil. Sift the flour into a large mixing bowl and add the baking powder and salt. Use your fingertips to rub the coconut oil into the flour until it resembles fine breadcrumbs, then add the water and mix together well to form a dough. Use your hands to gently push out the dough and line the pie dish with it. Carefully trim off the excess dough around the edges with a sharp knife. Set the dish aside.

2   To make the mushroom filling, heat up the tamari or water in a large saucepan set over a medium heat and add the onion and garlic. Cook for 3–4 minutes, until the onion starts to soften. Add the carrot and cook for 6–8 minutes, stirring occasionally, until it begins to soften. Add the vegetable stock, wine, dried thyme and chilli flakes and bring to the boil for 2–3 minutes. Reduce the heat, then add the mushrooms, nutritional yeast and seasoning. Cover partly with a lid and allow it to simmer gently for another 10–12 minutes, until cooked through. Stir occasionally to prevent it from burning.

3   While the mushrooms cook, prepare the sweet potato mash. Place the chopped sweet potatoes in a medium pot, cover with water and bring to the boil over a high heat for 2 3 minutes. Reduce the temperature to a medium heat, partly cover with a lid and simmer for 10–12 minutes, until the sweet potatoes can be easily sliced with a knife.

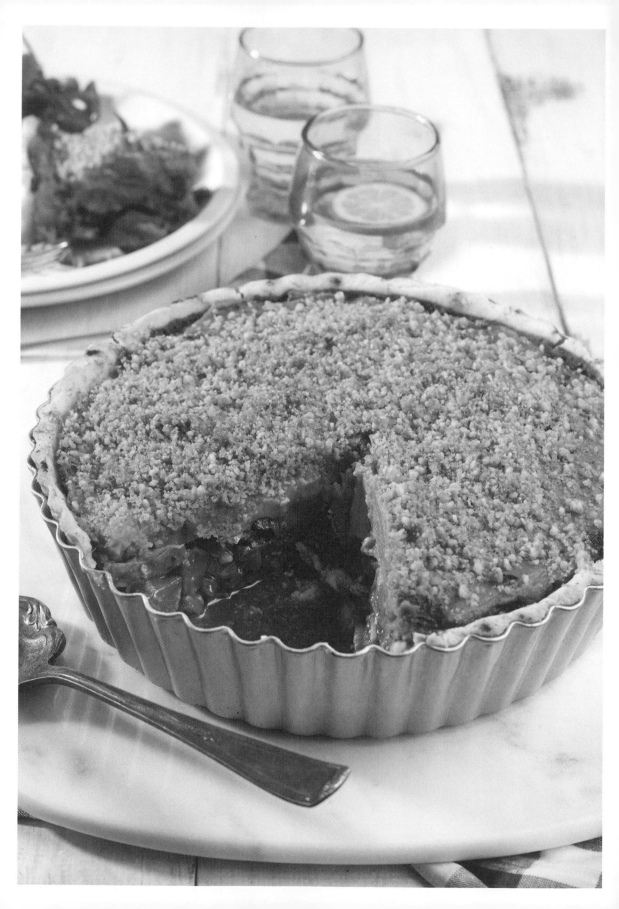

4   Drain the sweet potatoes and place in a blender or food processor. Add the nutritional yeast, if using, coconut oil, smoked paprika and seasoning and blend together until a smooth mash is formed. You may need to use some warm water to help it blend. Alternatively, place the potatoes back into the dry pot and mash thoroughly with a potato masher.

5   To make the pine nut Parmesan, place all the ingredients in a blender or food processor and blitz on a high speed until a crumbly mixture forms. Set aside.

6   Preheat the oven to 190°C.

7   To assemble the pie, pour the mushroom mixture into the pie dish lined with the crust. Top with the sweet potato mash, smoothing it evenly across the top of the mushrooms. Sprinkle the top of the sweet potato with the pine nut Parmesan and bake in the oven for 30–35 minutes, until golden.

8   Allow the pie to cool for 5 minutes before serving hot. Any leftovers can be stored in an airtight container in the fridge for three or four days.

Italian Herb Pizza with Sun-Dried Tomato and Basil Pesto and Cashew Cheese

SERVES 4 | PER SERVING: 639 CALORIES | 19.1G PROTEIN | 78.8G CARBS | 31G FAT

FOR THE PIZZA BASE:

250g white rice flour
(I recommend the Doves Farm brand)

2 tsp Italian dried herb blend

1 tsp xanthan gum

1 tsp gluten-free baking powder

sea salt and freshly ground black pepper

250ml water

2 tbsp coconut oil, melted, plus extra to grease

FOR THE CASHEW CHEESE:

130g raw unsalted cashews

2 garlic cloves, peeled

60ml water

3 tbsp nutritional yeast

2 tbsp fresh lemon juice

1 tbsp wholegrain mustard

FOR THE SUN-DRIED TOMATO AND BASIL PESTO:

55g sun-dried tomatoes

20g fresh basil leaves

2 garlic cloves, peeled

6–8 tbsp water, to blend

2 tbsp extra virgin olive oil (omit for a lower-calorie pesto)

2 tbsp pine nuts

1 tbsp nutritional yeast (optional)

1 tbsp fresh lemon juice

pinch of dried chilli flakes

PIZZA TOPPINGS:

70g white mushrooms, sliced

8–10 black or green olives, pitted and halved

1 red or yellow bell pepper, deseeded and finely sliced

½ ripe avocado, halved, stoned and sliced

ANTIOXIDANT-RICH   GOOD MOOD

MUSCLE-BUILDING   SLEEP-ENHANCING

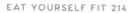

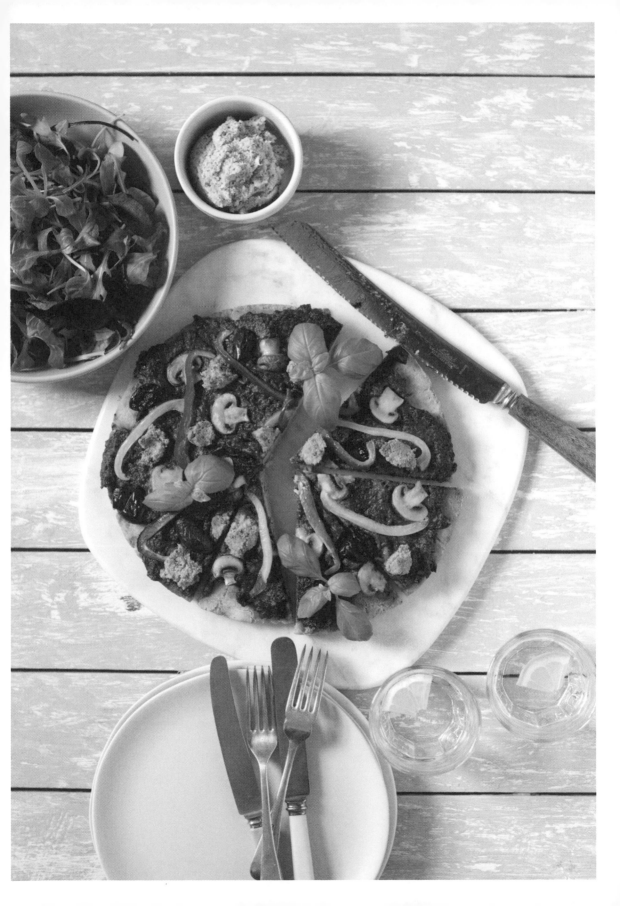

I don't think I've ever met a person who doesn't like pizza, although traditional pizza doesn't suit everyone and I certainly find it difficult to digest. This recipe uses rice flour to create a base that's soft and light on the inside and crispy on the outside. Topped with a sun-dried tomato and basil pesto, a creamy cashew cheese and some of my favourite vegetables, it's a very satisfying and filling alternative.

1 First soak the cashews in a bowl of cold water for 1 hour, then drain well.

2 Preheat the oven to 200°C. Lightly grease a 23cm round baking tin with coconut oil.

3 To make the base, sift the flour into a large mixing bowl and add the Italian herbs, xanthan gum, baking powder and seasoning. Mix together well. Add the water and stir to create a thick dough, then add the oil and mix together well. Transfer the dough to the greased baking tin and press it down evenly with your fingertips. Bake in the oven for 25–30 minutes, until the edges are starting to turn crisp and golden.

4 While the pizza base cooks, prepare the pesto. First use a sheet of kitchen paper to soak up any excess oil on the sun-dried tomatoes, then place all the ingredients in a blender or food processor and blend until smooth. Season to taste, then pour the pesto into a bowl and set aside.

5 Next, to make the cashew cheese, place the soaked and drained cashews into the blender or food processor with the rest of the ingredients and blend until smooth and creamy, stopping to scrape down the sides if necessary. Add extra water to help it blend if needed and season to taste with salt and pepper.

6 Remove the pizza base from the oven and spread with a thick layer of pesto, then top with the mushrooms, olives, pepper and avocado (or your choice of toppings). Drizzle on the cashew cheese, then place the pizza back in the oven for another 10–15 minutes, until the cashew cheese begins to turn golden.

7 Enjoy the pizza warm or cold. Any leftovers can be stored in a covered container in the fridge for three or four days.

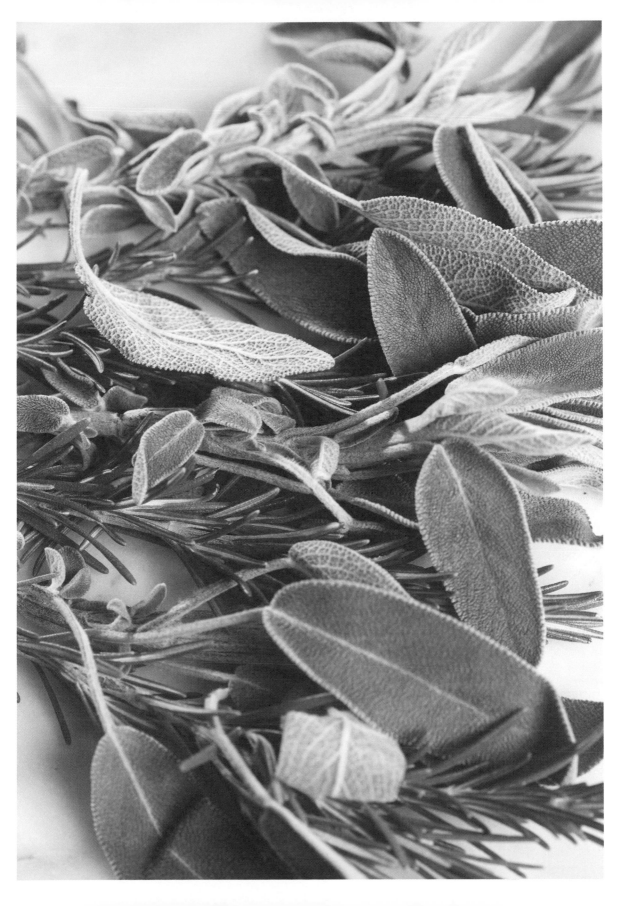

SNACK SMART

Fitness tip

If you get into the habit of choosing SMART SNACKS to munch on when hunger strikes between meals, a STRONG, lean, HEALTHY BODY becomes so much easier to achieve and maintain. Ditch the sugar and processed foods and whizz up one of the DELICIOUS DIPS in this section to enjoy with veggie sticks and seeded crackers, or impress your family and friends with your own homemade kale crisps.

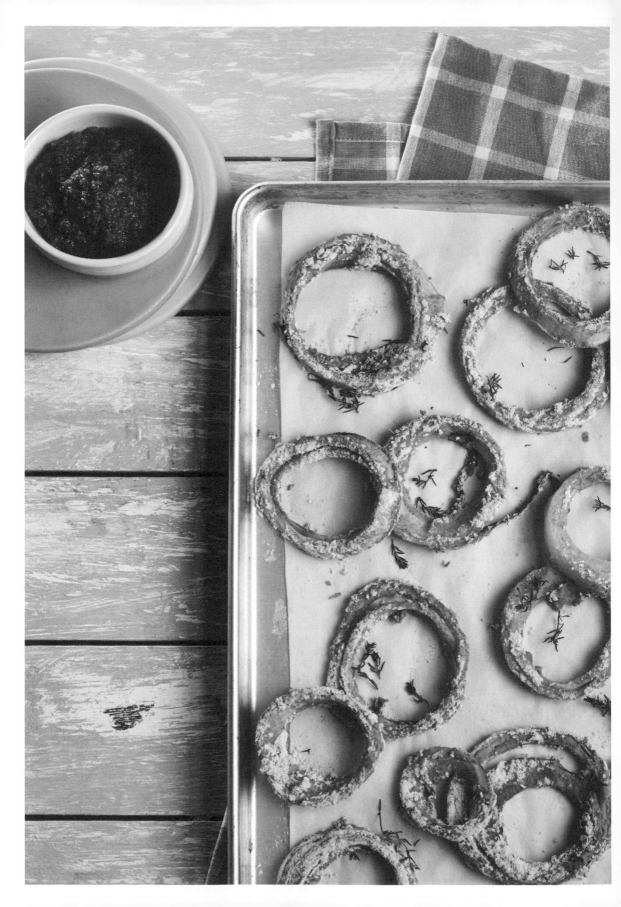

Crispy Baked Onion Rings with Sweet Chilli Sauce

SERVES 4 | PER SERVING: 270 CALORIES | 15.1G PROTEIN | 46.3G CARBS | 3.8G FAT

coconut oil, to grease

125ml water

120g chickpea flour
(gram flour)

6 tbsp nutritional yeast

2 tbsp ground cumin

1 tbsp garlic powder

2 tsp smoked paprika

pinch of cayenne pepper

4 medium red or white
onions, peeled and sliced
into rings

**FOR THE SWEET CHILLI
SAUCE:**

2 red bell peppers, deseeded
and roughly chopped

4 dates, pitted and chopped,
or 1 tbsp pure maple syrup
or honey

1 red chilli, deseeded and
chopped

1 garlic clove, peeled

1 tbsp fresh lime juice

1 tsp chopped fresh ginger

sea salt and freshly ground
black pepper

Crunchy onion rings and sweet chilli sauce get a low-calorie makeover in this healthy snack recipe, which uses chickpea flour and a selection of spices to coat the onion rings. They're always a big hit with family and friends and are the perfect pairing for this sugar-free sweet chilli sauce.

1   Preheat the oven to 200°C. Lightly grease two large baking trays with coconut oil or line with non-stick baking paper.

2   Mix the water and 30g of the chickpea flour in one bowl. Mix the remaining 90g chickpea flour with the nutritional yeast and spices in a separate bowl.

3   Submerge the onion rings in the water and flour mixture, then coat them well in the spice mixture. Lay them out on the baking tray and bake in the oven for 20–25 minutes, until golden brown and crisp.

4   Meanwhile, place all the ingredients for the sweet chilli sauce in a blender or food processor and blend on high speed for 30–40 seconds, until smooth.

5   Serve the onion rings with the sweet chilli sauce on the side. Any leftovers can be stored in a covered container in the fridge for four or five days.

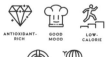

ANTIOXIDANT-RICH   GOOD MOOD   LOW-CALORIE

MUSCLE-BUILDING   SLEEP-ENHANCING

Cheesy Curried Kale Crunchies

SERVES 2 | PER SERVING: 171 CALORIES | 13.7G PROTEIN | 10G CARBS | 5.5G FAT

coconut oil, to grease

150g fresh kale

2 medium tomatoes,
roughly chopped

1 garlic clove, peeled

2 tbsp hulled hemp seeds

2 tbsp nutritional yeast

1 tbsp tamari

1 tbsp fresh lemon juice

2 tsp curry powder

2 tsp smoked paprika

1 tsp Cajun spices

pinch of cayenne pepper
(optional)

sea salt and freshly ground
black pepper

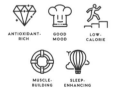

ANTIOXIDANT-RICH   GOOD MOOD   LOW-CALORIE

MUSCLE-BUILDING   SLEEP-ENHANCING

These cheesy curried kale crunches are the perfect healthy alternative to regular crisps. They're a crunchy and satisfying snack, low in carbs, fat and calories but high in protein, phytochemicals and essential good mood nutrients.

1   Preheat the oven to 180°C. Lightly grease two baking trays with coconut oil.

2   Prepare the kale by removing the tough stalks, ripping the leaves into smaller pieces and rinsing well. Gently pat dry with kitchen paper, transfer to a large mixing bowl and set aside.

3   Place the rest of the ingredients in a blender and blend until a thick, smooth sauce forms. Taste and adjust the seasoning as needed.

4   Pour the sauce on top of the kale and mix together well, ensuring the kale is well coated. Spread out the kale on the baking trays and dry it out in the oven with the door left slightly open. This should take 40–45 minutes, but keep an eye on the kale to ensure it doesn't burn and turn it over after 20 minutes to allow both sides to bake.

5   Serve warm or cold. Any leftovers can be stored in an airtight container for up to two days, but the kale is best eaten on the day it's made.

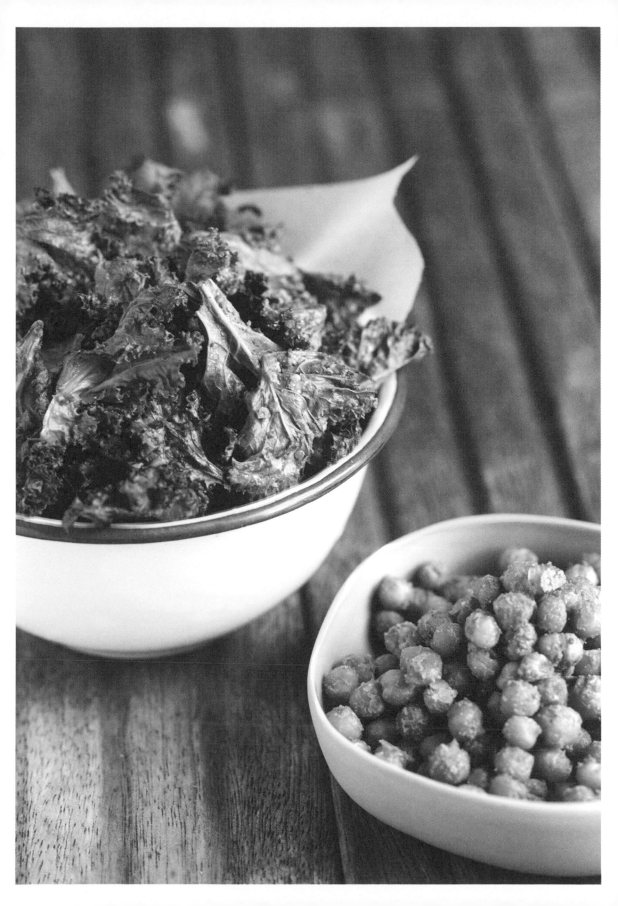

Spicy Roast Chickpea Bites

SERVES 2 | PER SERVING: 258 CALORIES | 13.7G PROTEIN | 34.5G CARBS | 8G FAT

1 x 400g tin of chickpeas, drained and rinsed

2 tbsp nutritional yeast

2 tsp coconut oil, melted

1–2 tsp smoked paprika

1 tsp ground cumin

1 tsp garlic powder

pinch of cayenne pepper (optional)

sea salt and freshly ground black pepper

ANTIOXIDANT-RICH   LOW-CALORIE

MUSCLE-BUILDING

Crispy, spicy and completely addictive, these chickpea bites are a great way to add more fibre and protein to your diet. If a strong and lean body is your goal, this is a super snack to munch on.

1 Preheat the oven to 190°C. Line a large baking tray with non-stick baking paper.

2 Pat the rinsed chickpeas dry with kitchen paper and place them in a large mixing bowl. Add the nutritional yeast, melted coconut oil, smoked paprika, cumin, garlic powder, cayenne pepper, if using, and seasoning. Toss together until the chickpeas are well coated.

3 Spread the chickpeas out on the baking tray and roast in the oven for 25–30 minutes, until they're crisp and golden. Stir the chickpeas or shake the tray every 10 minutes. Remove from the oven and allow the chickpeas to cool for 10 minutes to crisp up even more.

4 The chickpeas are best enjoyed on the day they're made, but can be stored in an airtight container in a cool, dry place for two or three days.

Omega-3 Superseed Crackers

SERVES 4–6 | PER SERVING: 287 CALORIES | 10.5G PROTEIN | 20G CARBS | 20.2G FAT

170g flaxseeds
160g whole chia seeds
500ml cold water
4 tbsp tamari
1 tsp garlic powder
sea salt and freshly ground
black pepper

GOOD MOOD   MUSCLE-BUILDING

SLEEP-ENHANCING

All the fibre and omega-3 goodness of flax and chia seeds packed into a crispy, lightly salted cracker. They're simple, nutritious and a healthier option than store-bought crackers. I enjoy them dipped into hummus (try my recipes on page 227 or page 228) or guacamole (page 129 or page 181).

1   Soak the seeds in the cold water and tamari for 1 hour to encourage them to stick together.
2   Preheat the oven to 180°C. Line two baking trays with non-stick baking paper.
3   Spread the soaked seeds out across the trays and ensure they're smooth and even, then sprinkle over the garlic powder and salt and pepper. Bake them in the oven for 45–50 minutes, until they are completely dried out.
4   Once fully dry, remove from the oven and allow them to cool for 15 minutes, then cut into crackers. Store in an airtight container in a cool, dry place for up to three days.

Garlic and Rosemary Bread

MAKES 1 LOAF | PER SERVING: 209 CALORIES | 3.4G PROTEIN | 43G CARBS | 2.3G FAT

2 garlic cloves, peeled

635g sweet potato, peeled and cut into quarters

475g rice flour, spelt flour or gluten-free all-purpose flour

1 tbsp milled flaxseeds

1 tbsp coconut oil, melted, plus extra for greasing

1 tsp dried rosemary

1 tsp dried parsley

1 tsp onion powder

1 tsp gluten-free baking powder

½ tsp gluten-free baking soda

pinch of sea salt

60ml water

1 tbsp sesame seeds

ENERGY-BOOSTING   GOOD MOOD

SLEEP-ENHANCING

The special key ingredient for creating texture and flavour in this bread is sweet potato. Using it means that you can really reduce the fat and oil content, making it a healthy and fibre-filled bread. I love the flavours of roast garlic and rosemary together in it, and it goes very well with my carrot, coconut and red lentil soup on page 160.

1   Preheat the oven to 190°C. Lightly grease a loaf tin with coconut oil or line with non-stick baking paper.

2   Place the garlic cloves in the tin and roast in the oven for 10–12 minutes, until lightly golden. Remove from the oven and set aside, but keep the oven on.

3   Steam the sweet potato for 8–10 minutes, until soft and easy to slice with a knife. Place the roast garlic and sweet potato in a blender or food processor and blend together into a smooth purée, using 3–4 tablespoons of water to help it blend if necessary.

4   In a large mixing bowl, combine the sweet potato and garlic purée with the flour, flaxseeds, melted coconut oil, rosemary, parsley, onion powder, baking powder, baking soda and a pinch of sea salt. Use your hands to knead the dough until the sweet potatoes are well combined.

5   Gradually add the water to the mixture to create a soft dough, which should be soft but not sticky or wet. Add more flour if it's too wet or more water if it's too dry and knead for another 3–4 minutes.

6   Transfer the dough to the prepared loaf tin and ensure the top is smooth and even without pressing down on it too much. Sprinkle the sesame seeds on top and bake in the oven for 30–35 minutes, until golden or a knife comes out clean when it's inserted in the middle.

7   Remove from the oven and allow the loaf to cool for 5 minutes before transferring to a wire rack and cooling for another 10 minutes. Serve warm with your choice of topping.

8   The bread can be stored in an airtight container in a cool, dry place for two or three days and can be frozen for up to three months.

Sun-Dried Tomato and Basil Hummus

SERVES 2–3 | PER SERVING: 198 CALORIES | 11.3G PROTEIN | 29G CARBS | 5.2G FAT

1 x 400g tin of chickpeas,
drained and rinsed

8–10 sun-dried tomato halves

1 large garlic clove, peeled

2 tbsp nutritional yeast
(optional but advised)

1 tbsp fresh lemon juice

1 tbsp tahini

1 tsp smoked paprika

pinch of cayenne pepper or
dried chilli flakes

sea salt and freshly ground
black pepper

3–4 tbsp unsweetened
almond milk

1 handful of fresh basil leaves

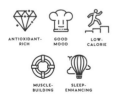

ANTIOXIDANT-RICH   GOOD MOOD   LOW-CALORIE

MUSCLE-BUILDING   SLEEP-ENHANCING

Sun-dried tomatoes always seem to make recipes taste a little bit more special, and they go extremely well with fresh, fragrant basil. This hummus tastes great as a dip, but I also love it on salads, in wraps and even stirred into soups.

1   Add the chickpeas to a food processor along with the sun-dried tomatoes, garlic, nutritional yeast, lemon juice, tahini, smoked paprika, cayenne pepper and seasoning. Slowly add the almond milk to help it blend and process until smooth and creamy or pulse to allow some texture to remain, stopping to scrape down the sides of the bowl if necessary. Add the basil and pulse again to combine. Taste and adjust the seasoning as needed.

2   Store any leftovers in an airtight container in the fridge for three or four days.

Sweet Potato and Spinach Hummus

SERVES 3–4 | PER SERVING: 164 CALORIES | 8.3G PROTEIN | 25.7G CARBS | 3.8G FAT

1 sweet potato, peeled and chopped into small chunks

1 x 400g tin of chickpeas, drained and rinsed

2 garlic cloves, peeled

juice of ½ lemon

2 tbsp nutritional yeast (optional)

1 tablespoon tahini

1 tsp Cajun spices

1 tsp smoked paprika

pinch of dried chilli flakes

dash of tamari

dash of unsweetened almond milk, to blend

sea salt and freshly ground black pepper

30g baby spinach

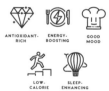

ANTIOXIDANT-RICH   ENERGY-BOOSTING   GOOD MOOD

LOW-CALORIE   SLEEP-ENHANCING

A tasty twist on traditional hummus, this low-calorie and oil-free dip is a great way to include more leafy greens in your diet. I love this hummus with raw carrot and cucumber sticks for a healthy snack or as a salad topping in place of creamy, calorific dressings.

1   In a medium-sized saucepan set over a medium to high heat, boil the sweet potato chunks in plenty of water for 10–12 minutes, until they're soft enough to slice into with a knife. Drain well and transfer to a blender or food processor. Add the chickpeas, garlic, lemon juice, nutritional yeast, if using, tahini, Cajun spices, smoked paprika, chilli flakes and a dash of tamari. Pulse to combine, using a little almond milk to help it blend if necessary.

2   Continue to pulse until the hummus reaches your desired texture, then taste and adjust the seasoning if necessary. Stir in the spinach, allowing it to wilt in the warmth.

3   Serve the hummus warm or allow it to chill in the fridge for 30 minutes before serving. The hummus can be stored in an airtight container in the fridge for up to four days.

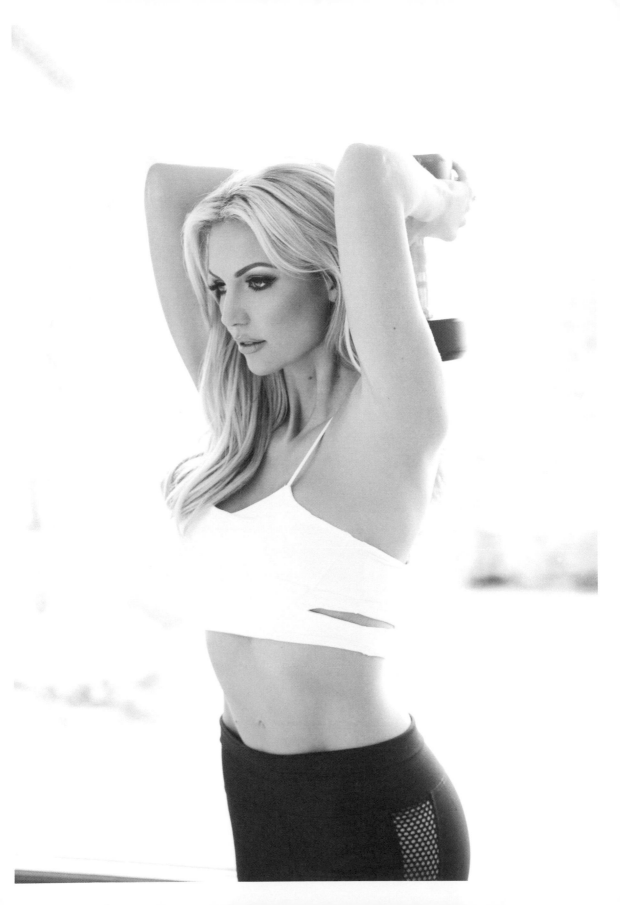

Roasted Red Pepper and Butter Bean Dip

SERVES 3–4 | PER SERVING: 78 CALORIES | 4.5G PROTEIN | 12.5G CARBS | 1.4G FAT

1 red pepper, deseeded and quartered

1 x 400g tin of butter beans, drained and rinsed

juice of ½ lemon

2 tbsp nutritional yeast (optional)

2 tsp smoked paprika

1 tsp tahini

dash of tamari

sea salt and freshly ground black pepper

GOOD MOOD   LOW-CALORIE

MUSCLE-BUILDING   SLEEP-ENHANCING

This low-fat, low-calorie dip packs in a lot of flavour. The sweet roasted pepper and smoked paprika work so well with the mellow, creamy butter beans. I love it as a healthy dip for raw vegetable sticks or my omega-3 superseed crackers on page 225.

1   Preheat the oven to 190°C. Line a small baking tray with non-stick baking paper.

2   Place the pepper on the tray and roast in the oven for 15–20 minutes, until its skin turns lightly golden brown.

3   Place the roasted pepper in a blender or food processor and add the butter beans, lemon juice, nutritional yeast, if using, smoked paprika, tahini, tamari and seasoning. Blend well until a smooth dip forms, adding a dash of water to help it blend if necessary.

4   Transfer to a bowl and serve with fresh vegetable sticks or enjoy on sandwiches, wraps and salads. Any leftovers can be stored in an airtight container in the fridge for three or four days.

Lime and Mint Avocado Salsa Boats

SERVES 2 | PER SERVING: 180 CALORIES | 2.7G PROTEIN | 13.5G CARBS | 14.9G FAT

1 ripe avocado, halved
and stoned

1 medium tomato, chopped

2 spring onions, chopped

1 handful of fresh mint leaves,
chopped

1 handful of fresh coriander
leaves, chopped

1 tbsp tamari

1 tbsp fresh lime juice

2 tsp brown rice vinegar

1 tsp smoked paprika, plus
a pinch to garnish

1 tsp coriander seeds or
ground coriander

½ tsp dried chilli flakes,
or to taste

sea salt and freshly ground
black pepper

ANTIOXIDANT-
RICH
LOW-
CALORIE

This makes a great snack, light meal or a simple starter for dinner parties. The zesty lime and refreshing mint work well with the cool creaminess of ripe avocado, and it's a fun way to enjoy one of the most perfect sources of healthy fat.

1   Scoop the flesh out of the avocado, setting the empty half shells aside. Chop the avocado into bite-sized pieces, then place in a mixing bowl with all the remaining ingredients. Mix together well, taking care not to mash the avocado. Taste and adjust the seasoning as needed.

2   Divide the filling between the avocado shells, sprinkle with a pinch of smoked paprika and serve. Any leftovers can be stored in a covered container in the fridge for up to two days, but it's best eaten as soon as possible so that the avocado doesn't brown.

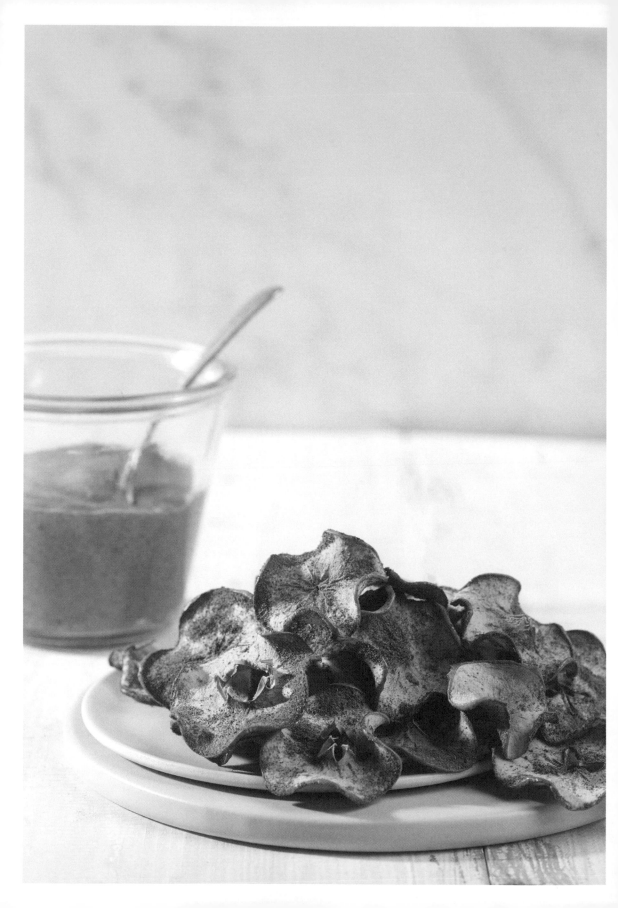

Spiced Apple Crisps

SERVES 2 | PER SERVING: 100 CALORIES | 0.5G PROTEIN | 27.2G CARBS | 0.3G FAT

2 firm apples, such as Braeburn or Pink Lady

2 tsp ground cinnamon

¼ tsp ground nutmeg

ANTIOXIDANT-RICH   GOOD MOOD

LOW-CALORIE   SLEEP-ENHANCING

Free from refined sugar, the natural sweetness of apple is enhanced by the warmth of ground cinnamon. Rich in antioxidants, try them dipped into almond butter for a satisfying snack that's perfect before bed to encourage restful sleep.

1   Preheat the oven to 125°C. Line one or two baking trays with non-stick baking paper.

2   Rinse and dry the apples, then use an apple corer to remove the cores and seeds. Using a mandolin, slice the apples very thinly. Place the apple slices in a large bowl and toss with the cinnamon and nutmeg to coat.

3   Spread the apple slices across the baking trays and bake in the oven for approximately 2 hours, until crunchy, flipping the slices halfway through to ensure they're evenly baked. Remove from the oven and allow the slices to cool before serving. They taste especially good dipped in nut or seed butter.

4   Store any leftovers in an airtight container for up to three days.

Chunky Monkey Peanut Butter Ice Cream

SERVES 2 | PER SERVING: 303 CALORIES | 6.5G PROTEIN | 42.7G CARBS | 14.6G FAT

65ml unsweetened almond milk or low-fat coconut milk

2 bananas, peeled, cut into chunks and frozen for at least 2 hours or overnight

3 dates, pitted and soaked in hot water for 5–10 minutes to soften

2 tsp vanilla extract, vanilla powder or vanilla bean paste

½ tsp ground cinnamon

½ tsp almond extract

pinch of ground nutmeg

6–8 drops of liquid stevia (optional)

2 tbsp smooth or crunchy peanut butter (try to buy an organic brand with no added sugar or palm oil)

TO SERVE:

4 medium-large strawberries, hulled and sliced

1 tbsp cacao nibs or dairy-free dark chocolate chips

1 tbsp raw walnut pieces

I've put this ice cream in the snacks section because it makes such a satisfying bite to eat, but it's so healthy and energy-boosting that you could also enjoy it for breakfast. Packed with natural energy from the dates and frozen banana and the healthy fats and protein of the peanut butter and walnuts, your friends and family won't believe that this delicious ice cream is so good for you.

1   Place the almond milk, frozen banana chunks, soaked and drained dates, vanilla, cinnamon, almond extract, nutmeg and stevia, if using, in a blender or food processor and blend on high for 2–3 minutes, until the mixture becomes smooth and resembles soft-serve ice cream. If it becomes too liquid, place it in the freezer for an hour to set. Transfer to a mixing bowl and use a spoon to swirl in the peanut butter.

2   Serve cold, topped with strawberries, cacao nibs or chocolate chips and raw walnut pieces. It can be made 2 hours in advance and stored in the freezer, but it's best eaten as soon as it's made.

ENERGY-BOOSTING   GOOD MOOD

SLEEP-ENHANCING

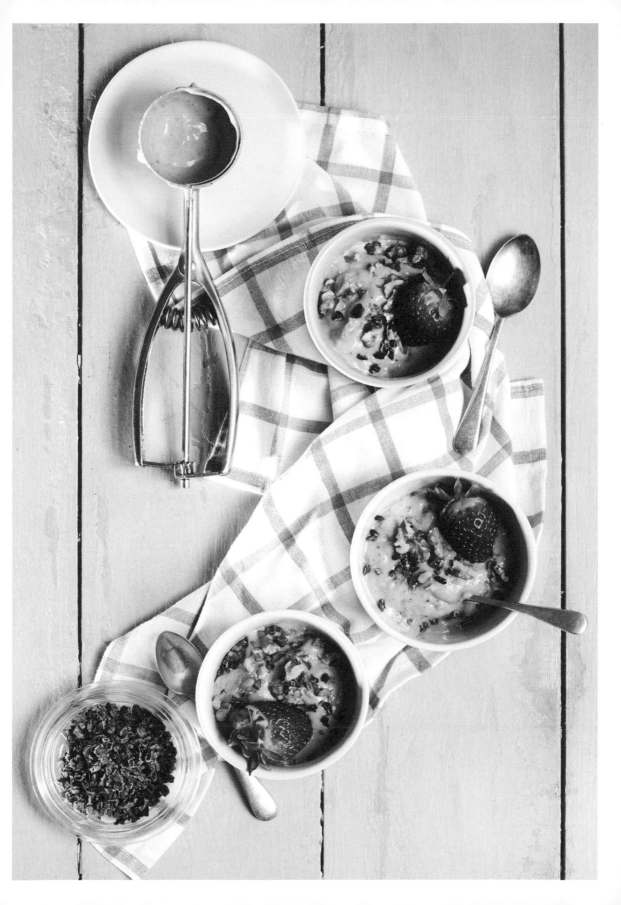

Chocolate Brownie Superfood Amazeballs

MAKES 16 BALLS | PER BALL: 103 CALORIES | 3G PROTEIN | 11.3G CARBS | 5.9G FAT

145g raw unsalted almonds

25g raw cacao powder or unsweetened cocoa powder

1 tsp ground cinnamon

1 tsp vanilla extract or powder

150g dates, pitted, chopped and soaked in hot water for 20 minutes to soften

2–3 tbsp water, to blend

3 tbsp cacao nibs or unsweetened dark chocolate chips

4–6 drops of liquid stevia (optional)

TO COAT:

4 tbsp raw cacao powder or unsweetened desiccated coconut

ANTIOXIDANT-RICH   ENERGY-BOOSTING

GOOD MOOD   MUSCLE-BUILDING

Healthy ingredients are blended and rolled into superfood brownie balls for an energising and filling snack. Dates, cinnamon and vanilla add natural sweetness, with some crunch from the raw almonds and heaps of antioxidants from the cacao powder.

1   Place the almonds in a food processor and process until coarsely ground. Add the cacao powder, cinnamon and vanilla and pulse again to combine. Add the soaked and drained dates and slowly add the water. Process until a thick, sticky dough has formed. Pulse in the cacao nibs and stevia, if using.

2   Roll pieces of the dough into small, tablespoon-sized balls. You can roll them in the cacao powder, coconut or any other toppings of your choice.

3   Place your brownie bites in a container in the refrigerator or freezer for at least 30 minutes, then serve chilled. Any leftovers can be stored in an airtight container in the fridge for four or five days.

Fitness Fudge Brownies

MAKES 4–6 BROWNIES | PER BROWNIE (SWEETENED WITH MAPLE SYRUP): 100 CALORIES

2.2G PROTEIN | 22.7G CARBS | 1G FAT

3 ripe medium bananas

45g raw cacao powder
or unsweetened dark
cocoa powder

2 tbsp pure maple syrup or
honey or 3–4 pitted, chopped
dates, to sweeten (optional)

1 tsp vanilla extract or powder

½ tsp gluten-free
baking powder

ANTIOXIDANT-RICH   ENERGY-BOOSTING   GOOD MOOD   LOW-CALORIE

These soft and rich chocolate fudge brownies are the perfect post-workout treat to refuel. Puréed banana creates the naturally sweet flavour and soft texture without the need for flour, fat or sugar. Cacao powder is rich in antioxidants and magnesium to help repair and protect your cells after exercise and prevent tight muscles.

1   Preheat the oven to 200°C. Line a 20cm square baking tin with non-stick baking paper.
2   Place the bananas in a blender or food processor and blend to a smooth purée. Transfer the bananas to a mixing bowl and fold in the cacao powder, then add the sweetener, if using, vanilla and baking powder. Mix together well until a thick batter forms.
3   Pour the batter into the prepared tin and bake in the oven for 15–18 minutes, until the top has darkened slightly and is firm to touch. The middle will still look soft. Remove from the oven and allow the brownies to cool for 10 minutes. They will set more in the middle as they cool.
4   Slice into brownies and serve. Any leftovers can be stored in an airtight container in the fridge for three or four days.

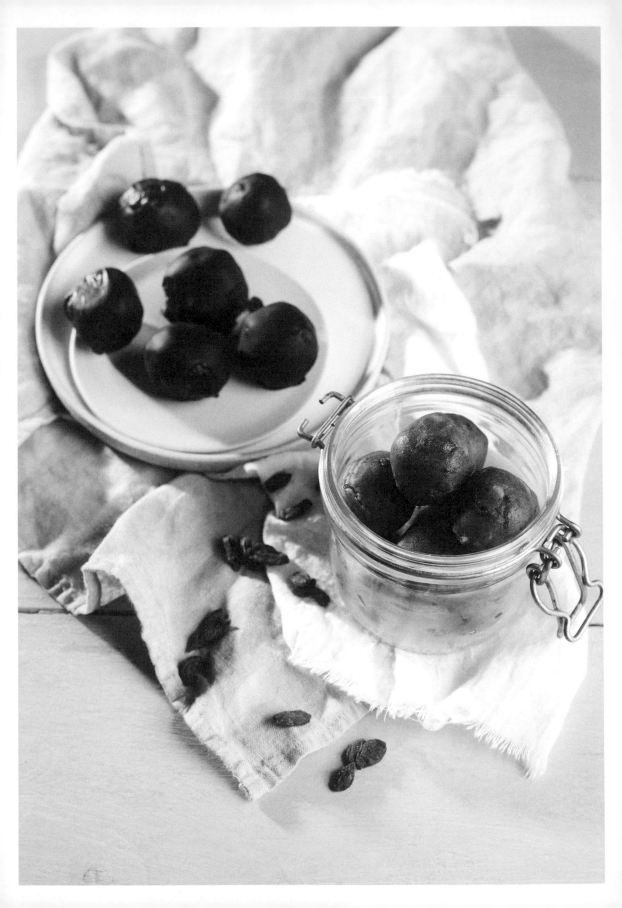

Peanut Butter and Goji Berry Protein Amazeballs

MAKES 15 BALLS | PER BALL: 54 CALORIES | 3.3G PROTEIN | 5.9G CARBS | 2.4G FAT

75g dates, pitted, chopped and soaked in hot water for 20 minutes to soften

2 scoops of Sunwarrior vanilla protein powder

4 tbsp smooth or crunchy peanut butter (look for organic peanut butter, free from added sugar and palm oil)

2 tbsp goji berries

2 tsp vanilla extract

1 tsp ground cinnamon (optional)

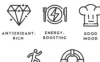

A great post-workout snack, breakfast on the go or guilt-free sweet treat when you fancy something tasty and satisfying. The goji berries add a pop of crunchy sweetness and help to boost the nutritional value of these balls even more. They're a rich source of antioxidant vitamins A and C, energy-boosting B vitamins and iron, plus magnesium, potassium and selenium.

1   Drain the soaked dates well and place them in a food processor or blender along with a splash of warm water. Blend until a smooth paste forms, adding more water if necessary.

2   Place the protein powder, peanut butter, goji berries, vanilla and cinnamon, if using, into a large mixing bowl and add 2 tablespoons of the date paste. Mix the ingredients together well until a thick dough forms. Taste at this point and add more vanilla or cinnamon if desired.

3   Roll the mixture into even-sized balls and lay them out on a piece of non-stick baking paper. Place the balls in the fridge to set for 30 minutes, then serve chilled. Leftovers can be stored in an airtight container in the fridge for up to three days.

CHEAT CLEAN: DESSERTS AND SWEET TREATS

Fitness tip

It would be crazy to go through life without
treats, and I firmly believe that it's important
to reward HARD WORK and HEALTHY LIVING.
Although all these desserts and sweet treats
are FREE from DAIRY, GLUTEN and REFINED
SUGAR, they're not intended for everyday
eating, as many are ENERGY RICH. I love to
make one of these delicious desserts when
I really feel like I've earned it. The best
time for indulging is actually straight after
a workout, when your body requires QUICK
ENERGY and burns up food faster.

SOS Chocolate Bark

MAKES 20 PIECES | PER SERVING: 140 CALORIES | 3.4G PROTEIN | 11.7G CARBS | 9.5G FAT

30g raw hazelnuts, skinned and chopped

30g slivered almonds

20g unsweetened coconut flakes

110g coconut oil

80g pure maple syrup or honey

45g raw cacao powder or unsweetened dark cocoa powder

2 tsp vanilla extract or powder

2 tbsp goji berries

2 tbsp dried apricots, chopped

1 tbsp pistachios, chopped

ANTIOXIDANT-RICH   ENERGY-BOOSTING

GOOD MOOD   LOW-CALORIE

I have been struck with a dark chocolate craving on more than one occasion, generally late at night. So what's a girl to do? I came up with this recipe for simple and quick homemade chocolate bark to make when the shops are closed and only chocolate will do. I thought it would be apt to name it SOS chocolate, as it has saved the day plenty of times. It's delicious topped with your favourite nuts, seeds and dried fruit. I like to use toasted coconut flakes, slivered almonds, chopped hazelnuts, pistachios, goji berries and dried apricots.

1   Preheat the oven to 190°C.

2   Spread out the hazelnuts, slivered almonds and coconut flakes on a baking tray. Toast them in the oven for 10 minutes, until golden. Set aside, then line the tray with non-stick baking paper.

3   Melt the coconut oil in a saucepan set over a medium heat, then add the maple syrup, cacao and vanilla. Stir until a smooth chocolate sauce forms, then mix in half of the nuts and coconut flakes until well distributed.

4   Pour the chocolate mixture into the lined tray and smooth it across the top with a spatula.

5   Sprinkle with the remaining toasted nuts and coconut plus the goji berries, apricots and pistachios. Place the tray in the freezer on a flat surface to set for 30 minutes.

6   Remove the tray from the freezer and slice or break the chocolate bark into pieces. Serve chilled. The bark is best stored in the fridge or freezer and eaten straightaway, as it begins to melt quite quickly at room temperature.

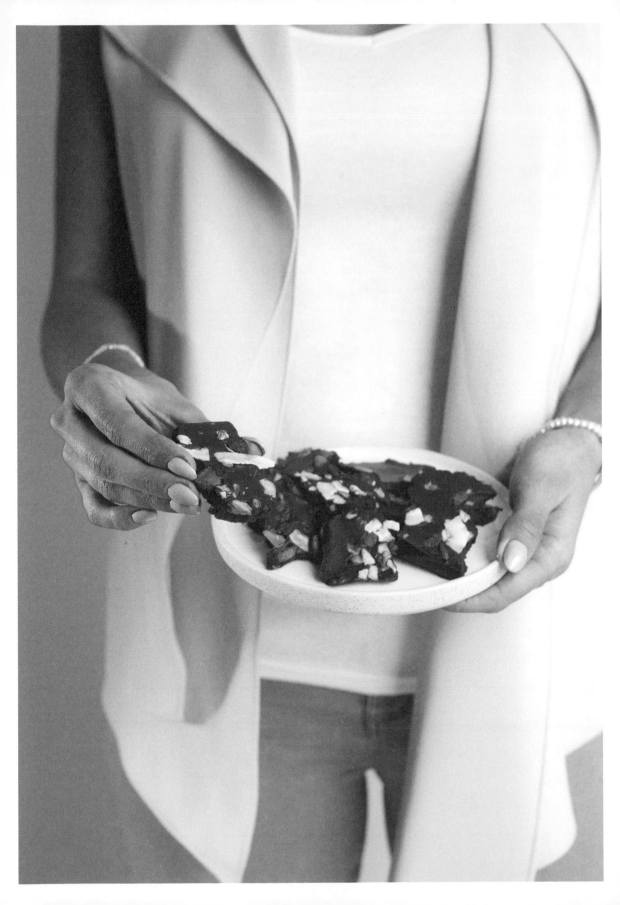

Salted Caramel Bliss Balls

MAKES 20 BALLS | PER BALL: 156 CALORIES | 2.1G PROTEIN | 25G CARBS | 6.1G FAT

FOR THE SALTED CARAMEL FILLING:

225g dates, pitted and soaked in hot water for 20 minutes to soften

1 tsp vanilla extract or powder

½ tsp sea salt, plus extra for sprinkling on top

60g smooth almond butter

FOR THE CHOCOLATE SHELL:

260g dark chocolate (at least 70–85% cacao content)

1 tbsp coconut oil

ANTIOXIDANT-RICH   ENERGY-BOOSTING

GOOD MOOD   LOW-CALORIE

Bliss balls by name and bliss balls by nature! These salted caramel, almond butter and chocolate truffles make a delicious and decadent treat. Make a big batch to keep in the fridge for a sneaky sweet treat or to share with loved ones. Either way, they're a guaranteed hit.

1   Line a large baking tray with non-stick baking paper.

2   Place the soaked and drained dates in a food processor and blend until they form a sticky dough or thick paste. Use a small splash of warm water to help it blend and stop to scrape down the sides if necessary. Add the vanilla and salt and pulse to combine.

3   Use a tablespoon to scoop out the mixture and form it into about 20 small balls. Place the balls on the prepared tray, then put the tray in the freezer for 30 minutes to set. Once the caramel has set, use a teaspoon to drizzle almond butter across the tops of all the truffles. Place back into the freezer for another 15–20 minutes.

4   Meanwhile, fill a small or medium saucepan one-third full with water and set a medium bowl on top to form a double boiler, making sure the bottom of the bowl doesn't touch the water. Bring the water to the boil, then reduce to a simmer and place the chocolate and coconut oil in the bowl, stirring gently as it melts together.

5   Remove the tray of truffles from the freezer. Use a fork to quickly immerse each truffle in the chocolate sauce, ensuring it's covered evenly. Shake off any excess chocolate and place each truffle back on the tray.

6   Place the tray back in the freezer to set again for 30 minutes and serve chilled. Store the truffles in an airtight container in the fridge for up to a week.

Pecan Pie Truffles

MAKES 10 TRUFFLES | PER TRUFFLE: 161 CALORIES | 2.5G PROTEIN | 13.8G CARBS | 11.9G FAT

150g raw pecan halves

75g dates, pitted and soaked in hot water for 20 minutes to soften

30g raw cacao powder or unsweetened dark cocoa powder, plus extra for coating

3 tbsp pure maple syrup or honey

1 tbsp smooth unsalted almond butter

1 tsp ground cinnamon

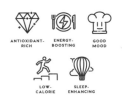

ANTIOXIDANT-RICH   ENERGY-BOOSTING   GOOD MOOD

LOW-CALORIE   SLEEP-ENHANCING

These rich pecan and cacao truffles take just minutes to make and are the perfect way to satisfy a craving for a guilt-free sweet nibble or a late-night chocolate treat when you're getting cosy on the sofa.

1 Preheat the oven to 190°C.
2 Spread the pecans out on a baking tray and bake in the oven for 10 minutes, until lightly toasted. Set aside to cool.
3 Place the toasted pecans, soaked and drained dates, cacao powder, maple syrup, almond butter and cinnamon in a blender or food processor. Blend until the mixture is well combined into a thick dough.
4 Place 3–4 tablespoons of cacao powder in a shallow bowl. Roll the truffle mixture into 10 balls, then roll the balls in the cacao powder until fully covered.
5 Place in the fridge to chill until ready to serve. Store in an airtight container in the fridge for four or five days.

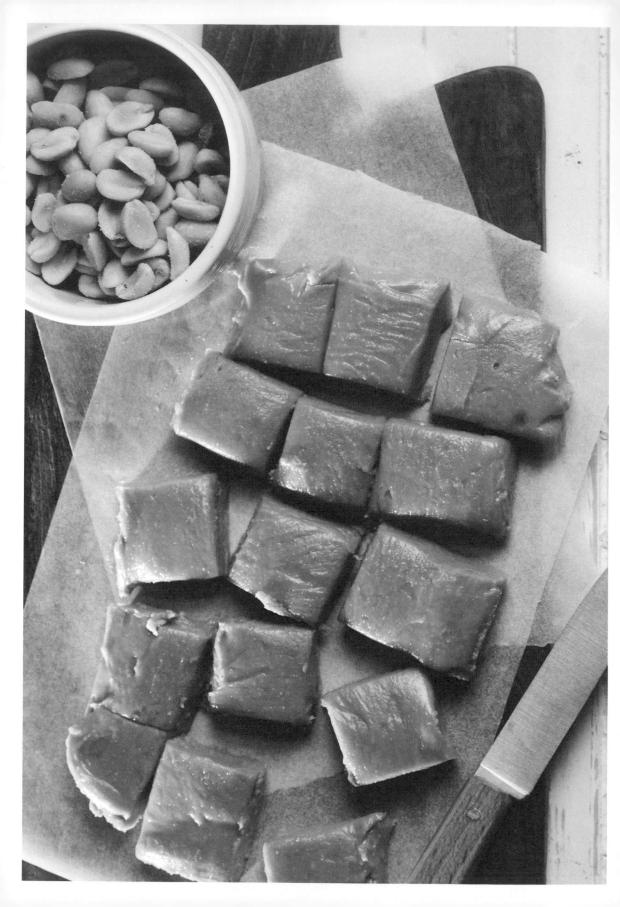

Vanilla Peanut Butter Fudge

MAKES 10 PIECES | PER PIECE: 142 CALORIES | 4.2G PROTEIN | 5.5G CARBS | 12.4G FAT

190g smooth peanut butter

2 tbsp coconut oil, softened

1 tbsp pure maple syrup
or honey

1 tsp vanilla extract or powder

pinch of sea salt

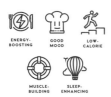

ENERGY-
BOOSTING   GOOD
MOOD   LOW-
CALORIE

MUSCLE-
BUILDING   SLEEP-
ENHANCING

This is the most deliciously creamy and decadent sweet fudge, made with just five ingredients. I like to make a batch of it when friends are coming over, and nobody believes that it's free from refined sugar and made from natural ingredients. But be warned, it can be difficult to stop at just one square!

1   Combine all the ingredients in a small bowl and mix until smooth. Transfer the batter to a medium-sized dish lined with non-stick baking paper and smooth the top with a spatula. Place the dish in the freezer and allow to set for 20–30 minutes, or until firm.

2   Cut into squares and serve immediately. Always serve chilled. Leftovers can be kept in an airtight container in the fridge for two or three days or in the freezer for up to three months.

Chewy Cranberry and Pecan Cookies

MAKES 8 COOKIES | PER COOKIE: 306 CALORIES | 3.7G PROTEIN | 36G CARBS | 18.8G FAT

180g unsweetened
dried cranberries

110g raw pecans

60g gluten-free rolled oats

55g dates, pitted and chopped

40g unsweetened
desiccated coconut

4 tbsp milled flaxseeds

2 tbsp coconut oil, melted,
plus extra to grease

2 tbsp pure maple syrup
or honey

3 tsp ground cinnamon

2 tsp vanilla extract or powder

ANTIOXIDANT-RICH   ENERGY-BOOSTING

GOOD MOOD   SLEEP-ENHANCING

Crispy, chewy and lightly spiced, with a pop of sweetness from the cranberries, these wholesome cookies are simple to make and taste delicious. Everything gets mixed together in the food processor and then baked, meaning minimal mess and clearing up afterwards.

1   Preheat the oven to 190°C. Lightly grease a baking tray with coconut oil or line it with non-stick baking paper.
2   Place all the ingredients in a blender or food processor and blend until the mixture forms a sticky dough. Roll into 8 balls and place on the tray, pressing down gently to form a disc. Alternatively, use a cookie cutter to form the shapes.
3   Bake in the oven for 15–20 minutes, until golden and firm to touch. Remove from the oven and let the cookies cool for a few minutes before carefully transferring them to a wire cooling rack. Store the cookies in an airtight container in a cool place for three or four days.

Raspberry and Vanilla Shortbread

MAKES 10 SLICES | PER SLICE: 315 CALORIES | 6.2G PROTEIN | 29.5G CARBS | 19.5G FAT

170g gluten-free rolled oats

120g pure maple syrup

110g coconut oil, melted, plus extra for greasing

85g ground almonds

2 tsp vanilla extract or powder

12 fresh raspberries, chopped

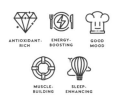

ANTIOXIDANT-RICH   ENERGY-BOOSTING   GOOD MOOD

MUSCLE-BUILDING   SLEEP-ENHANCING

Growing up, classic shortbread was my favourite baked treat to make. I loved the sweet and buttery texture. This version is just as rich and crumbly, thanks to the combination of oats and ground almonds, and the delightful duo of raspberry and vanilla makes these biscuits an absolute must-try.

1   Preheat the oven to 190°C. Lightly grease a 16cm x 22cm x 5cm baking tin with coconut oil or line with non-stick baking paper.

2   Place the oats in a blender or food processor and blend until a fine flour forms. Place the flour in a large mixing bowl with the maple syrup, melted coconut oil, ground almonds and vanilla and stir well until a thick dough forms. Add the chopped raspberries and ensure they're evenly distributed. Transfer the mixture to the baking tray and press down firmly, making sure it's smooth and even.

3   Bake in the oven for 25–30 minutes, until the shortbread turns golden brown and crisp on top. Remove from the oven and allow to cool on a wire rack for 10 minutes before cutting into slices. The shortbread is best eaten on the day it's made, but leftovers can be stored in an airtight container in the fridge for two or three days.

Hazelnut Butter Cookies

MAKES 10 COOKIES | PER COOKIE: 189 CALORIES | 4.1G PROTEIN | 14.9G CARBS | 13.1G FAT

coconut oil, to grease

2 tbsp milled flaxseeds

4 tbsp cold water

250g crunchy hazelnut butter
(almond or peanut butter can
also be used)

160g pure maple syrup
or honey

2 level tsp gluten-free
baking powder

2 tsp ground cinnamon

2 tsp vanilla extract or powder

4 tbsp chopped hazelnuts

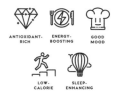

ANTIOXIDANT-RICH   ENERGY-BOOSTING   GOOD MOOD

LOW-CALORIE   SLEEP-ENHANCING

Easy, quick and delicious cookies made with wholesome ingredients and full of fibre, protein and heart-healthy fats. Crisp on the outside and soft and chewy on the inside, I love how simple they are to make and bake.

1   Preheat the oven to 180°C. Lightly grease a baking tray with coconut oil or line with non-stick baking paper.

2   First, make the flax 'egg' by mixing the milled flaxseeds with the cold water in a small bowl until well combined. Set aside to thicken up for 10 minutes.

3   Mix all the remaining ingredients except the chopped hazelnuts in a larger bowl, then add the flax 'egg'. Stir until the almond butter and maple syrup are well combined and they form a sticky dough. Use a tablespoon to divide out the dough to form the cookies, gently pressing down each one onto the baking tray. The mixture may be too sticky to even roll into balls first, so just smooth them out with the back of the spoon. Scatter the chopped hazelnuts on top, pressing them in slightly.

4   Bake in the oven for 20–25 minutes, until they're firm to touch and turning brown on top. Allow to cool on a wire rack for 10 minutes before serving. The cookies can be kept for up to three days in an airtight container.

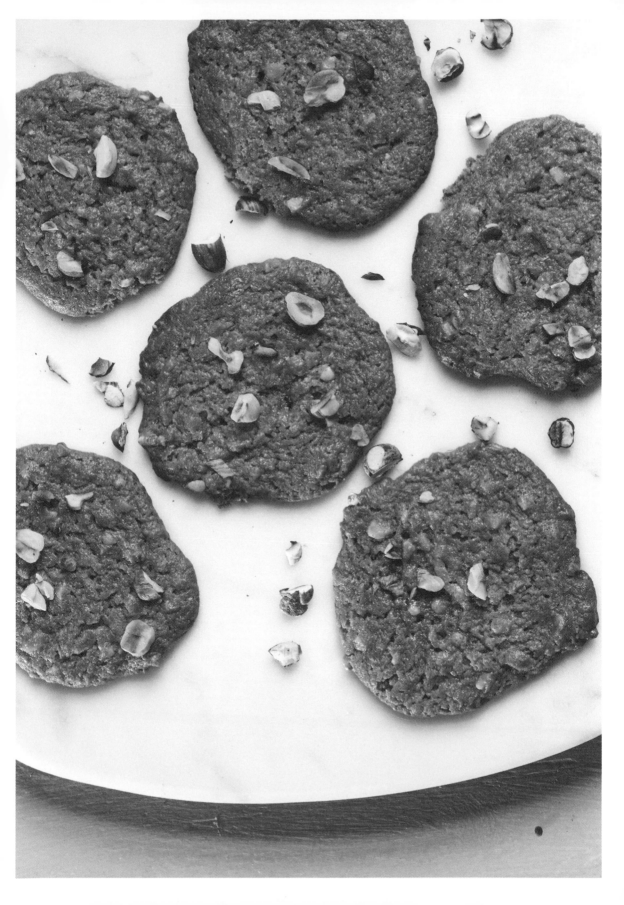

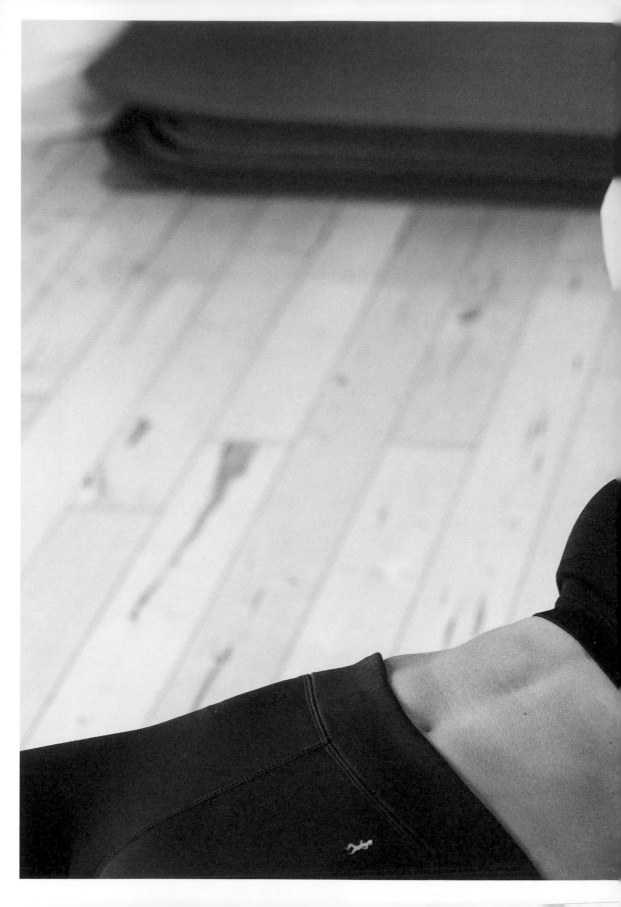

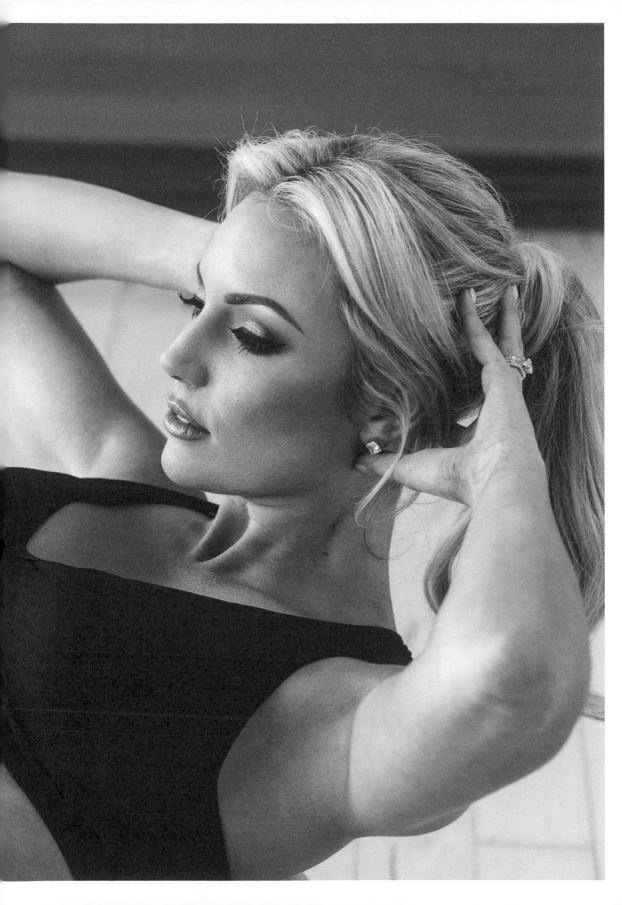

Zesty Lemon and Coconut Cream Slices

MAKES 12 SLICES | PER SLICE: 341 CALORIES | 6.7G PROTEIN | 25.2G CARBS | 26.3G FAT

FOR THE CRUST:

150g dates, pitted and soaked in hot water for 20 minutes to soften

130g raw unsalted almonds, chopped

100g raw pecans, chopped

40g unsweetened desiccated coconut

1 tbsp coconut oil, melted

pinch of ground cinnamon

FOR THE FILLING:

1 x 400ml tin of full-fat coconut milk, chilled overnight in the fridge

190g cashews, soaked in water for 30 minutes

100g pure maple syrup or honey

¼ ripe avocado

2 tbsp coconut oil, melted

1 tsp vanilla extract or powder

½ tsp ground turmeric (optional, for a yellow colour)

zest and juice of 2 lemons

toasted coconut flakes, to decorate

I've always loved citrus desserts, and lemon drizzle cake was a favourite when I was growing up. These lemon and coconut cream slices are a deliciously cool and zesty option for lemon lovers and the perfect treat for warm summer days.

1 Line a 20cm square baking tin with non-stick baking paper.

2 Place the soaked and drained dates, nuts, desiccated coconut, melted coconut oil and cinnamon in a food processor. Blend for 2 minutes, until the mixture is crumbly but sticks together. Use a dash of water to help it blend if necessary. Press the base mixture evenly into the bottom of the lined tin and set aside.

3 To make the filling, first carefully open the tin of chilled coconut milk without shaking it and scoop out the hardened coconut cream, which should have separated from the coconut water. Place it in a blender or food processor and add the soaked and drained cashews, maple syrup, avocado, melted coconut oil, vanilla, turmeric and the lemon juice and zest (but set some zest aside for sprinkling over the top later). Blend together until smooth and creamy, using a dash of water to help it blend if necessary.

4 Pour the filling evenly across the base and smooth the top with a spatula, then scatter over some toasted coconut flakes. Place the dish in the freezer to set for 30 minutes, until firm to touch.

5 Remove from the freezer, top with a sprinkle of lemon zest, cut into slices and serve chilled. Any leftovers can be stored in an airtight container in the fridge for three or four days.

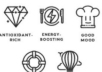

ANTIOXIDANT-RICH   ENERGY-BOOSTING   GOOD MOOD

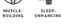

MUSCLE-BUILDING   SLEEP-ENHANCING

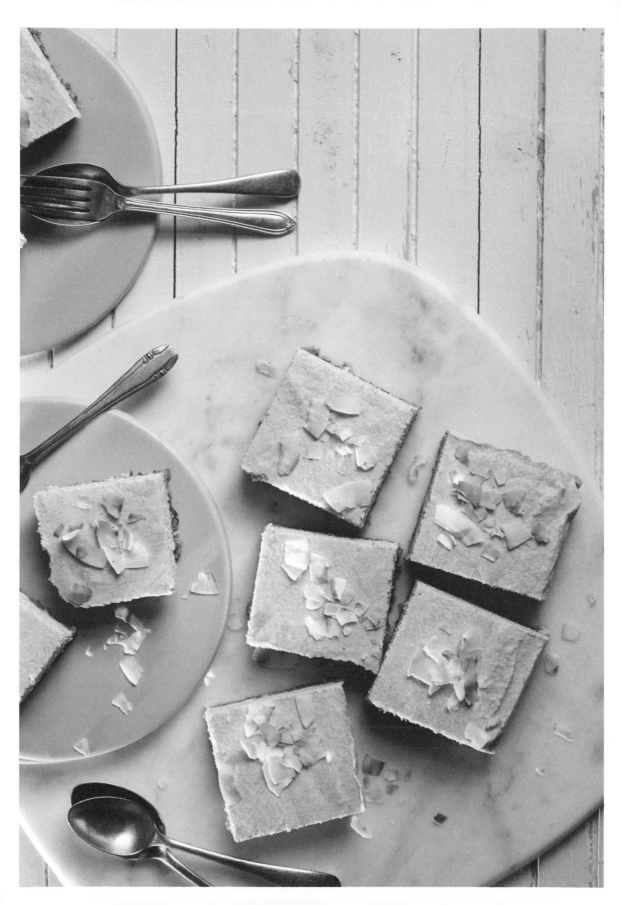

No-Bake Mars Bars

MAKES 4–6 BARS | PER BAR: 369 CALORIES | 4.7G PROTEIN | 44.5G CARBS | 22.3G FAT

FOR THE BASE:

110g raw pecans, chopped

115g dates, pitted and soaked in warm water for 20 minutes to soften

1 tsp vanilla extract or powder

FOR THE MIDDLE CARAMEL LAYER:

150g dates, pitted and soaked in warm water for 20 minutes to soften

2 tbsp smooth almond butter

2 tbsp pure maple syrup or honey

1 tsp vanilla extract or powder

2–3 tbsp warm water, to blend

FOR THE TOP CHOCOLATE LAYER:

2 tbsp coconut oil

2 tbsp raw cacao powder or unsweetened dark cocoa powder

2 tbsp pure maple syrup or honey

1 tbsp almond butter or tahini

1 tsp vanilla extract or powder

These gooey, rich and chocolaty Mars Bars are by far my most popular and most requested recipe. It's that irresistible combination of a thick, rich base, a squidgy caramel centre and a melt-in-the-mouth chocolate topping. A total crowd pleaser, you simply can't go wrong with a tray of healthier Mars Bars!

1   To make the base, place the pecans, soaked and drained dates and vanilla extract in a food processor or blender and blend until the mixture forms a dough that sticks together. You may need to add the ingredients bit by bit so as not to overwhelm the machine. Press the mixture down firmly in a medium baking tray or silicone tray, ensuring it's smooth and even.

2   Next, make the caramel layer. Place all the ingredients in a food processor or blender, adding the water if necessary to help it blend into a smooth, thick caramel sauce. Spread the caramel layer across the base and place it in the freezer to set for 15–20 minutes.

3   To make the chocolate layer, gently melt the coconut oil in a small saucepan set over a low-medium heat and add the cacao powder, maple syrup, almond butter and vanilla extract, stirring well until a thick, smooth chocolate sauce forms. Spread a layer of the chocolate sauce across the top of the caramel layer and place it back in the freezer to set for 25–30 minutes.

4   Once set and firm to touch, use a sharp knife to carefully slice the mixture into bars. Keep refrigerated until ready to serve and serve chilled. These bars will keep in the fridge in a covered container for up to three days and can be frozen for up to three months.

ANTIOXIDANT-RICH   ENERGY-BOOSTING

GOOD MOOD

Healthier Snickers Bars

MAKES 6 LARGE OR 12 SMALL BARS | PER SMALL BAR: 195 CALORIES | 4G PROTEIN

15.9G CARBS | 13.9G FAT

FOR THE NOUGAT LAYER:

125g smooth almond butter

2 tbsp pure maple syrup
or honey

1 tbsp coconut flour

**FOR THE CARAMEL
FILLING:**

110g dates, pitted and soaked
in hot water for 20 minutes
to soften

80ml water

1 tbsp coconut oil, melted

1 tsp vanilla extract or powder

pinch of sea salt

35g dry-roasted
unsalted peanuts

**FOR THE DARK
CHOCOLATE COATING:**

4 tbsp coconut oil

5 tbsp raw cacao powder
or unsweetened dark
cocoa powder

2 tbsp pure maple syrup
or honey

1 tbsp smooth almond butter

1 tsp vanilla extract or powder

ANTIOXIDANT-   ENERGY-
RICH   BOOSTING

GOOD
MOOD

Love traditional Snickers bars? It's great to know that you can whip up a healthier version at home whenever you fancy this peanut-packed treat. These homemade bars are naturally sweetened and made from nutrient-rich ingredients.

1   Line a large rectangular baking tray with non-stick baking paper.
2   Make the nougat layer by placing the almond butter, maple syrup and coconut flour in a medium bowl and mixing together well to combine. Press the mixture into the baking tray to create a rectangle about 1.25cm thick. Freeze for 30 minutes to set.
3   To make the caramel filling, place the soaked and drained dates, water, melted coconut oil, vanilla and salt in a blender or food processor and blend at high speed until smooth and creamy. Use a dash of water to help it blend if necessary and scrape down the sides of the blender a couple of times.
4   Take the nougat layer from the freezer and spread about half of the date caramel filling evenly across the top, smoothing it with a spatula. You may have some caramel left over, as a larger batch needs to be made to achieve a smooth caramel, but it works well as a dip for fresh fruit. Distribute the peanuts across the top of the caramel layer and gently press them down into it. Place the tray back into the freezer to set for at least 30 minutes.
5   To make the chocolate coating, melt the coconut oil in a medium saucepan set over a low-medium heat, then add the cacao powder, maple syrup, almond butter and vanilla. Stir until smooth.
6   Remove the tray from the freezer and slice into 6 full-size bars or 12 smaller bars. Use a tablespoon to spread the chocolate sauce over the tops and sides of each bar, then pick them up to coat the bottom too. Gently place the bars back onto the tray and return them to the freezer to set for another 20 minutes.
7   Store the bars in the fridge or freezer, depending on how firm you like them, and always serve chilled, as they begin to melt at room temperature. They can be stored in an airtight container in the fridge for up to a week.

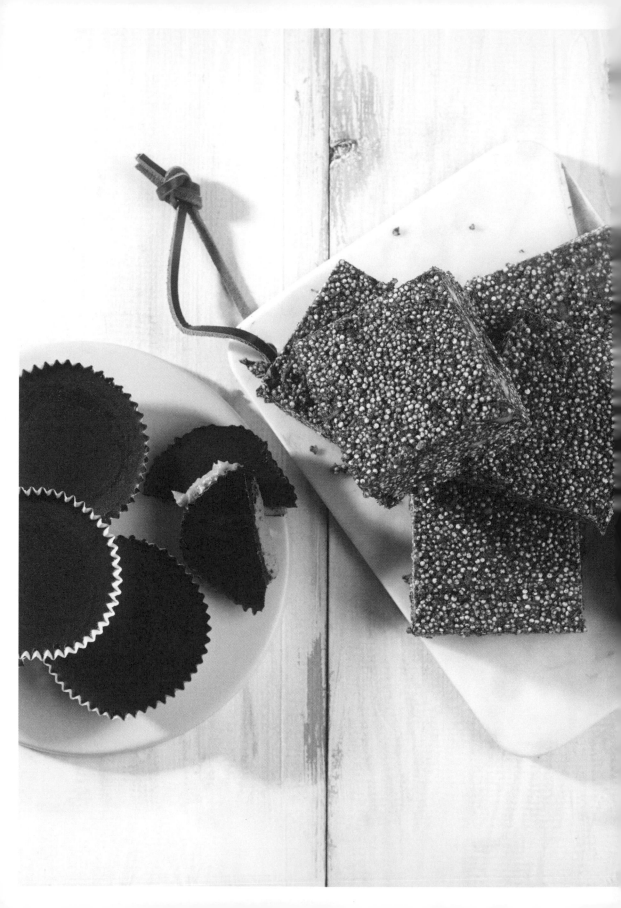

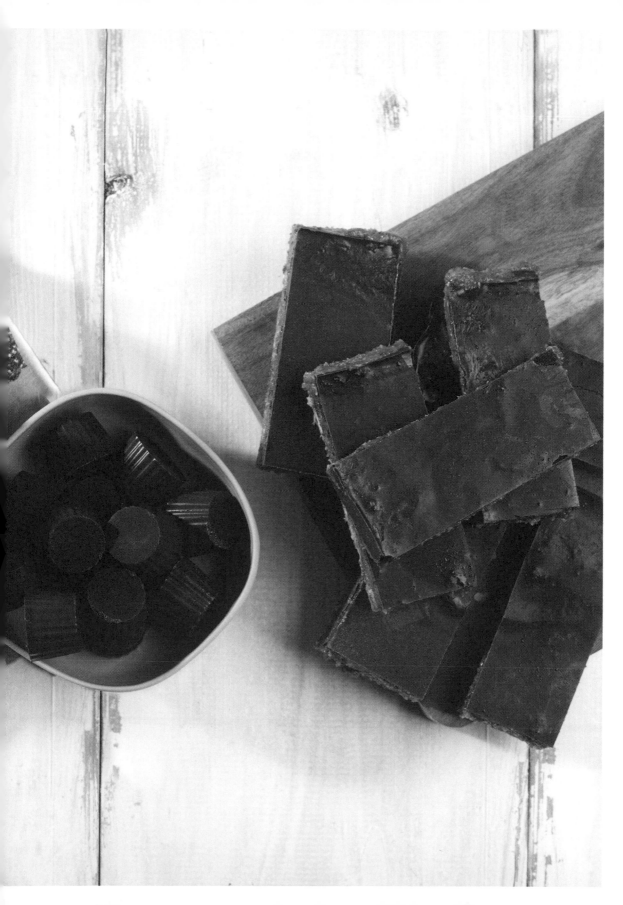

Fruit and Nut Quinoa Pop Bars

MAKES 12 BARS | PER BAR: 268 CALORIES | 5.1G PROTEIN | 23.9G CARBS, | 17.7G FAT

425g quinoa

220g coconut oil, melted

85g raw cacao powder
or unsweetened dark
cocoa powder

80g pure maple syrup
or honey

125ml unsweetened
almond milk

1 tsp vanilla extract

55g hazelnuts, raw or toasted,
chopped

35g raisins

20g unsweetened desiccated
coconut

3 tbsp cacao nibs or
unsweetened dark
chocolate chips

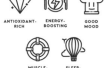

ANTIOXIDANT- ENERGY-   GOOD
RICH   BOOSTING MOOD

MUSCLE-   SLEEP-
BUILDING ENHANCING

I gently toast dry quinoa to help create these no-bake fruit and nut chocolate bars, as it adds a wonderful crunch and a warm, toasty flavour. They go particularly well with a frothy almond milk cappuccino.

1   First make the quinoa pops. Place a large saucepan over a medium heat and warm it up until it's hot. Add the quinoa in small amounts, stirring continuously so that it doesn't burn, until it pops and turns lightly golden brown. Keep adding the quinoa until the whole quantity has been popped and is lightly toasted. The quinoa grains won't open up or change shape in the way that popcorn does. Once all the quinoa has been toasted, set it aside.

2   Pour the melted coconut oil into a large mixing bowl and add the cacao powder, whisking until smooth. Add the maple syrup, followed by the almond milk and vanilla, continuing to whisk until the mixture turns silky and smooth. Stir in the quinoa pops, hazelnuts, raisins, desiccated coconut and cacao nibs and mix together well.

3   Pour the mixture onto a large baking tray lined with non-stick baking paper and spread it evenly with a spatula. Place the tray in the freezer to set for 30–40 minutes, then remove and cut into bars or squares. Store the bars in an airtight container in the fridge for six or seven days and always serve chilled.

Chocolate Peanut Butter Cups

MAKES 20 CUPS | PER CUP: 112 CALORIES | 2G PROTEIN | 6.5G CARBS | 9.3G FAT

FOR THE CHOCOLATE CUPS:

110g coconut oil, melted

45g raw cacao powder or unsweetened dark cocoa powder

100g pure maple syrup

1 tbsp smooth peanut butter (optional)

FOR THE PEANUT BUTTER FILLING:

125g smooth, creamy peanut butter (look for an organic brand free from added sugar and palm oil)

1 tsp vanilla extract or powder

1 tsp ground cinnamon (optional)

The most heavenly treat for all the peanut butter aficionados out there, these simple chocolate peanut butter cups are as good as any sweet snack gets. Smooth, rich and melt-in-the-mouth delicious.

1   Lay out 20 small cupcake cases on a large tray.
2   In a small bowl, combine the melted coconut oil and cacao powder until smooth, then stir in the maple syrup and the peanut butter, if using, until smooth and creamy.
3   To make the filling, mix together the peanut butter, vanilla and cinnamon in a separate bowl.
4   Pour a thin layer of chocolate sauce into the bottom of each cupcake case. Place in the freezer for 10 minutes to set, then remove from the freezer and divide the peanut butter filling between the cups. Pour the remaining chocolate sauce on top and place back in the freezer to set for 30 minutes.
5   Serve chilled and store in the fridge, as these cups will melt quite quickly at room temperature. Keep them in an airtight container in the fridge for up to a week.

Chocolate Fudge Cake with Raspberry Vanilla Cream

SERVES 6 | PER SERVING: 856 CALORIES | 10.6G PROTEIN | 128.8G CARBS | 36.5G FAT

320g gluten-free all-purpose white flour

320g coconut sugar

80g raw cacao powder or unsweetened dark cocoa powder

2 tsp gluten-free baking powder

½ tsp salt

375ml warm water

140g coconut oil, melted, plus extra to grease

2 tsp apple cider vinegar

2 tsp vanilla extract or powder

FOR THE RASPBERRY VANILLA CREAM:

3 x 400ml tins of full-fat coconut milk, chilled overnight in the fridge

100g fresh raspberries

1 vanilla pod, split in half lengthways and seeds scraped out, or 3 tsp vanilla extract

6–8 drops of liquid stevia, to sweeten (optional)

ANTIOXIDANT-RICH   ENERGY-BOOSTING

A soft, rich and indulgent chocolate fudge cake, perfect for birthdays and special occasions. Free from refined sugar, gluten and dairy, it tastes truly decadent with the raspberry vanilla cream. I love to surprise friends and family on their birthday with this cake, created for everyone to enjoy.

1   Preheat the oven to 190°C. Lightly grease 2 x 20cm cake tins with coconut oil, or use three small tins to create a three-tier cake, as pictured.

2   Sift the flour into a large mixing bowl, then add the coconut sugar, cacao powder, baking powder and salt. Mix it all together, ensuring the ingredients are well blended. Add the warm water, melted coconut oil, apple cider vinegar and vanilla extract, mixing until the wet and dry ingredients are well combined into a cake batter.

3   Divide the batter between the greased cake tins and bake in the oven for 25–30 minutes, until a knife comes out clean from the centre of the cake. Remove the cake tins from the oven and leave to cool for a few minutes before gently turning the cakes out onto a wire rack to cool completely.

4   Make the raspberry vanilla cream by gently opening the tins of chilled coconut milk without shaking them. The cream should have separated from the coconut water. Spoon the solid coconut cream into a blender and add most of the raspberries (save a handful to decorate the cake), the vanilla and the liquid stevia, if using. Blend until smooth and pink. Taste and add more vanilla or stevia if desired.

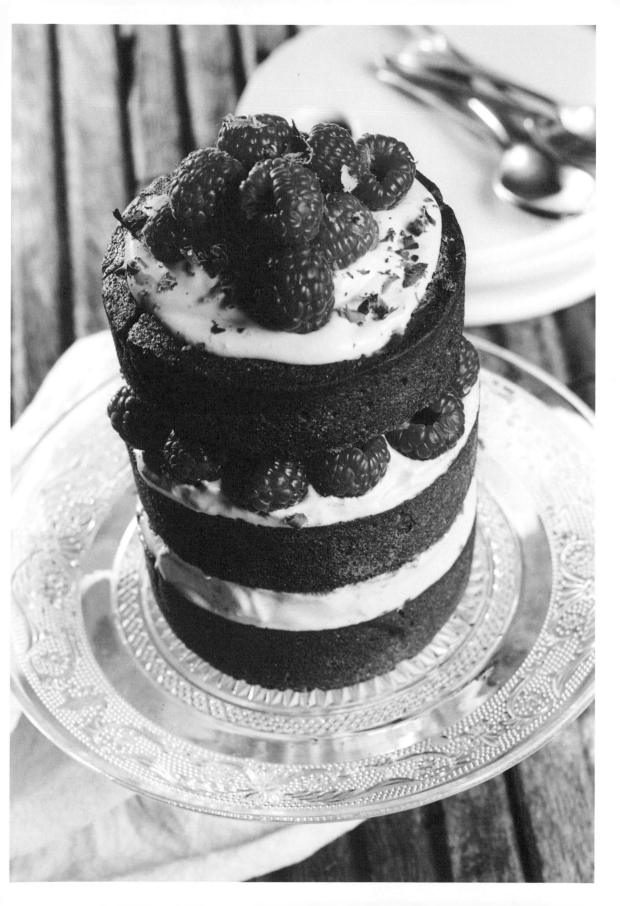

5 The cake must be fully cooled before you spread on the icing, as it will melt in any warmth. Place one of the cakes on a serving plate and spread a thick layer of icing across the middle, leaving a 2.5cm rim clear from the edges to allow for it to spread out more when you put the second cake on top. Add the top layer of sponge and spread the rest of the icing across the top of the cake.

6 Decorate with the reserved raspberries and a sprinkle of cacao powder. Leftovers must be stored in an airtight container in the fridge to keep the icing cool, and it will keep for up to three days.

Almond Swirl Fudge Brownies

MAKES 9 BROWNIES | PER BROWNIE: 243 CALORIES | 2.7G PROTEIN | 36.4G CARBS | 10.6G FAT

160g gluten-free flour

160g coconut sugar

50g raw cacao powder
or unsweetened dark
cocoa powder

1 tbsp milled chia seeds
or flaxseeds

1 tsp gluten-free
baking powder

1 tsp vanilla extract or powder

185ml warm water

70g coconut oil, melted,
plus extra for greasing

1 tsp apple cider vinegar

5–6 tsp smooth almond butter

ANTIOXIDANT-   ENERGY-
RICH   BOOSTING

GOOD
MOOD

These soft, rich fudge brownies are free from gluten and refined sugar
and make the most deliciously decadent treat. I love adding in the
almond butter swirl for an unusual twist, but you can leave it out if
you prefer, as they're just as tasty without it.

1   Preheat the oven to 190°C. Lightly grease an 18cm x 23cm or
    20cm square baking tin with coconut oil or line it with non-stick
    baking paper.

2   Sift the flour into a large mixing bowl and add the coconut sugar,
    cacao powder, chia or flaxseeds, baking powder and vanilla. Mix
    together to blend the ingredients well. Pour in the warm water
    and stir to form a thick batter, then add the melted coconut oil and
    apple cider vinegar and mix together.

3   Pour the batter into the prepared baking tin and smooth the top
    with a spatula. Use a teaspoon to gently swirl the almond butter
    across the top of the brownie batter.

4   Bake in the oven for 25–28 minutes, until it begins to turn crisp
    around the edges and a knife comes cleanly out of the centre of the
    mixture. Remove from the oven and allow the brownies to cool
    for 10–15 minutes before cutting into squares. Serve warm or
    cool. Any leftovers will keep in an airtight container in the fridge
    for five or six days.

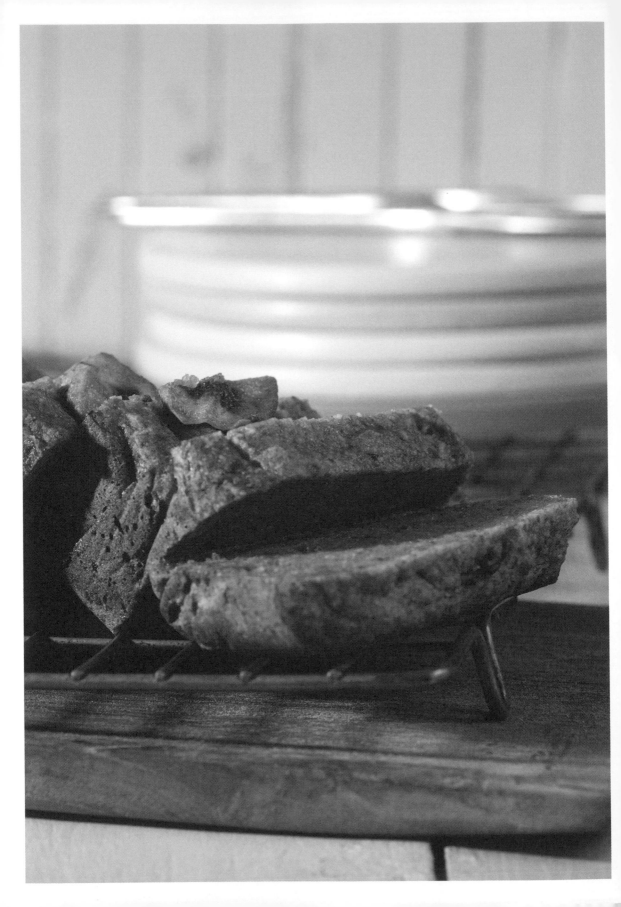

Banana Cake

MAKES 8 SLICES | PER SERVING: 308 CALORIES | 5.6G PROTEIN | 55.3G CARBS | 8.9G FAT

4 tbsp milled chia seeds

8 tbsp cold water

coconut oil, to grease

4½ ripe bananas

240g pure maple syrup
or honey

2 tsp vanilla extract or powder

200g white rice flour or
gluten-free all-purpose flour

100g ground almonds

2–3 tsp ground cinnamon

1 tsp gluten-free
baking powder

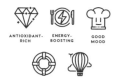

ANTIOXIDANT-
RICH   ENERGY-
BOOSTING   GOOD
MOOD

MUSCLE-
BUILDING   SLEEP-
ENHANCING

This delicious cake came about because, like many people, I had a bunch of bananas in the house that were a little too soft and ripe for eating, but I couldn't justify throwing them out. So they helped to make the most fudgy, dense and moist banana cake instead. The bananas act as a fantastic natural sweetener and binder for the mixture along with the chia seeds, which means you don't need to use any form of oil.

1   Start by placing the milled chia seeds in a small bowl, adding the water and mixing well. Set aside to allow the mixture to thicken.
2   Preheat the oven to 190°C. Lightly grease a loaf tin withd coconut oil or line with non-stick baking paper.
3   Place 4 bananas in a blender or food processor with the maple syrup, vanilla extract and chia mixture and blend until smooth. Cut the remaining ½ banana into slices.
4   Put the flour, ground almonds, cinnamon and baking powder in a bowl and mix well, then add the banana mixture. Mix everything together until a thick batter forms.
5   Transfer the batter to the loaf tin, smoothing the top. Decorate with the sliced banana and bake in the oven for 50–55 minutes, until the banana slices caramelise, the top turns golden brown and a knife comes out clean when inserted into the centre of the loaf.
6   Allow the loaf to cool on a wire rack for 10 minutes before slicing and serving. The loaf will keep for two or three days in an airtight container in the fridge.

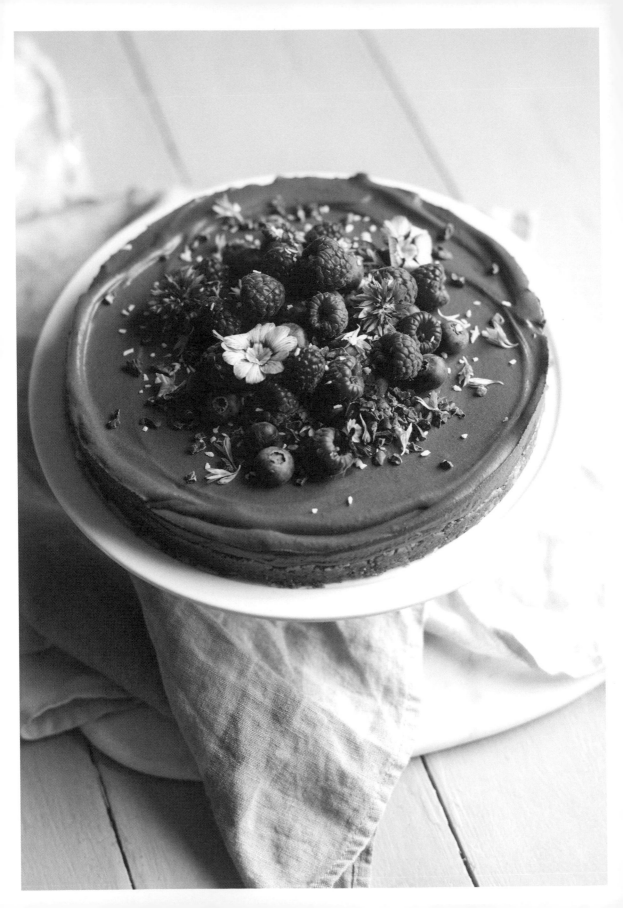

Chocolate Cheesecake

SERVES 6 | PER SERVING: 423 CALORIES | 5.5G PROTEIN | 42.7G CARBS | 28.8G FAT

FOR THE BASE:

150g dates, pitted and soaked for 20 minutes in hot water to soften

100g raw unsalted pecans

2 tbsp unsweetened desiccated coconut

2 tbsp smooth or crunchy almond butter

1 tbsp coconut oil, melted

2 tsp vanilla extract or powder

FOR THE CHEESECAKE FILLING:

2 x 400ml tins of full-fat coconut milk, chilled overnight in the fridge

6 tbsp raw cacao powder or unsweetened dark cocoa powder

6 tbsp pure maple syrup or honey

3 tsp vanilla extract or powder

½ ripe avocado, halved and stoned

1 tbsp coconut oil, melted

1–2 tbsp unsweetened almond milk, to blend

70g mixed fresh berries, to decorate

I made this rich, decadent and creamy chocolate cheesecake for my family on Christmas Day last year and it was a huge hit. It tastes just like the real thing, but uses healthier ingredients, free from refined sugar, gluten and dairy. It's so easy to make and keeps very well in the fridge.

1 To make the base, place the soaked and drained dates, pecans, desiccated coconut, almond butter, melted coconut oil and vanilla in a food processor fitted with an S blade. Process for 2–3 minutes, until a thick, sticky dough has formed. Press the base mixture into the bottom of a 20cm circular springform tin or silicone cake pan, ensuring the top is smooth and even.

2 To make the cheesecake filling, carefully open the tins of coconut milk without shaking them. The coconut cream should have separated from the coconut water and set in the fridge. Spoon out 6 tablespoons of thick coconut cream into a blender or food processor. Add the cacao powder, maple syrup, vanilla, avocado and melted coconut oil. Blend into a smooth, thick mixture, using a dash of almond milk to help it blend if needed.

3 Pour the cheesecake filling on top of the prepared base and smooth the top with a spatula to ensure it's even. Place the cheesecake into the freezer to set for 30–45 minutes, then remove from the freezer, top with fresh berries, slice into pieces and serve chilled.

4 The cheesecake can be stored in an airtight container in the fridge for three or four days.

ANTIOXIDANT-RICH   ENERGY-BOOSTING

GOOD MOOD   MUSCLE-BUILDING

Mini Toffee Cheesecakes

MAKES 7 | PER CHEESECAKE: 516 CALORIES | 11.1G PROTEIN | 46.3G CARBS | 36G FAT

FOR THE BASE:

150g dates, pitted and soaked
in hot water for 20 minutes
to soften

140g raw unsalted almonds
or walnuts

1–2 tsp ground cinnamon

1 tsp vanilla extract or powder

FOR THE CHEESECAKE
FILLING:

1 x 400ml tin of full-fat
coconut milk, chilled
overnight in the fridge

210g raw unsalted cashew
nuts, soaked in cold water for
15 minutes and drained

165g pure maple syrup
or honey

70g coconut oil, melted

1 tsp vanilla extract or powder

FOR THE TOFFEE SAUCE:

150g dates, pitted and soaked
for 20 minutes in hot water
to soften

1 tbsp tahini

1 tsp vanilla extract or powder

pinch of sea salt

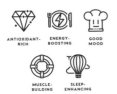

ANTIOXIDANT-   ENERGY-   GOOD
RICH   BOOSTING   MOOD

MUSCLE-   SLEEP-
BUILDING   ENHANCING

Creamy, silky miniature cheesecakes flavoured with toffee and vanilla, all on top of a chewy base. When I first made these at home to test the recipe, my husband polished them off in well under an hour. Always a good sign of a delicious dessert!

1 To make the base, drain the soaked dates well and place them in a food processor with the almonds, cinnamon and vanilla. Blend them together until a sticky dough forms. You should be able to stick the mixture together between your fingers. Use a tablespoon to divide the mixture evenly between the wells of a muffin tin (you should aim to make around 7 cheesecakes), pressing down gently on the mixture to help it stick together and making sure the tops are smooth and even.

2 To make the cheesecake filling, first carefully open the tin of chilled coconut milk without shaking it. The thick coconut cream should have separated from the coconut water. Spoon it out into a blender or food processor. Add the drained cashews, maple syrup, melted coconut oil and vanilla. Blend together until the mixture is smooth and creamy. Divide the filling between the bases in the muffin tray and make sure they're smooth across the top.

3 To make the toffee sauce, drain the soaked dates and place them in a blender with the tahini, vanilla and salt. Use a splash of warm water to help it blend into a smooth sauce. Stop and scrape down the sides of the blender if necessary. Use a teaspoon to place a dollop of toffee sauce on the centre of each cheesecake, smoothing it across the top.

4 Place the entire tray into the freezer to set for at least 2 hours. Remove from the freezer when ready to serve and use a blunt knife to ease the edges of the cheesecakes out from the tin, then pop them out. The cheesecakes are best eaten on the day they're made, but they can be stored in an airtight container in the fridge for up to two days.

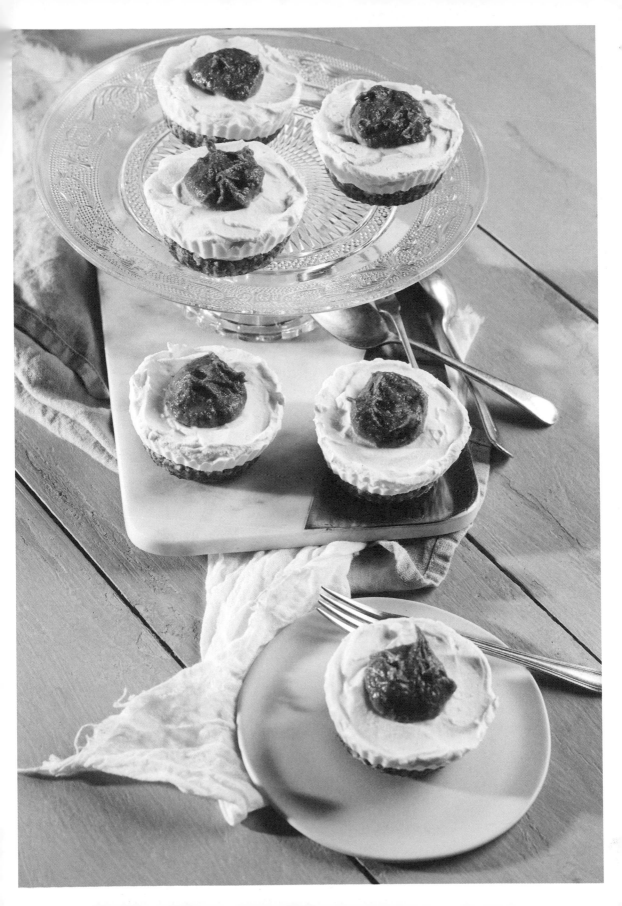

Sticky Toffee Pudding

SERVES 6 | PER SERVING: 717 CALORIES | 8.2G PROTEIN | 82.4G CARBS | 43G FAT

80g raw pecans

375ml unsweetened
almond milk

200g dates, pitted
and chopped

½ tsp gluten-free baking soda

75g coconut sugar

55g coconut oil, at room
temperature, plus extra
to grease

155g white rice flour or
gluten-free self-raising flour

1 tsp ground cinnamon

½ tsp ground ginger

pinch of ground nutmeg

FOR THE TOFFEE SAUCE:

160g pure maple syrup

125g smooth unsalted
almond butter

70g coconut oil

2 tsp vanilla extract or powder

pinch of sea salt

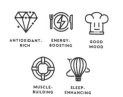

ANTIOXIDANT-RICH   ENERGY-BOOSTING   GOOD MOOD

MUSCLE-BUILDING   SLEEP-ENHANCING

An all-time favourite pudding complete with a sticky, sweet toffee sauce, but made with healthier ingredients. I've added fragrant spices and crunchy toasted pecans for extra texture.

1   Preheat the oven to 190°C. Lightly grease a 23cm pie dish with coconut oil or line with non-stick baking paper.

2   Spread out the pecans on a small baking tray and toast them in the oven for 8–10 minutes, until golden. Roughly chop them and set aside.

3   In a medium saucepan set over a medium-high heat, bring the almond milk to the boil. Add the chopped dates and reduce the heat to low for 1 minute, then remove from the heat and mix in the baking soda, allowing it to fizz slightly.

4   In a large mixing bowl, use a hand-held whisk or electric whisk to whisk together the coconut sugar and coconut oil until they're as smooth as possible. Add the almond milk and date mixture and combine well, then add the flour, cinnamon, ginger, nutmeg and toasted pecans to the mixing bowl and mix together until combined.

5   Transfer the sponge batter to the prepared pie dish, spreading it out evenly. Bake in the oven for 25–30 minutes, until the cake is firm but spongy to touch. Remove from the oven and allow it to cool for 10–15 minutes before slicing and serving.

6   While the cake bakes, make the toffee sauce. Add all the ingredients to a small saucepan set over a medium-low heat and whisk together for about 3 minutes, until all the ingredients have melted together into a smooth sauce. To make it even smoother, blend it at high speed in a blender for 30–40 seconds.

7   Serve the warm sauce over a slice of sticky toffee sponge. Any leftovers can be stored in an airtight container in the fridge for three or four days.

Apple, Pear and Pecan Crumble with Vanilla Whip

SERVES 10 | PER SERVING WITH VANILLA WHIP: 421 CALORIES

4.1G PROTEIN | 56G CARBS | 22.6G FAT

4 medium-large apples, peeled, cored and thinly sliced (I like to use Pink Lady)

4 medium-large ripe pears, peeled, cored and thinly sliced

50g coconut sugar

60ml water

3 tbsp cornstarch or arrowroot starch

2 tbsp fresh lemon juice

2 tsp ground cinnamon

1 tsp grated fresh ginger (optional)

½ tsp ground nutmeg

FOR THE CRUMBLE TOPPING:

145g coconut sugar

120g coconut oil, melted, plus extra to grease

90g gluten-free porridge oats

70g brown or white rice flour

55g ground almonds

50g pecans, chopped

1 tsp ground cinnamon

FOR THE VANILLA WHIP:

2 x 400ml tins of full-fat coconut milk, chilled overnight in the fridge

2 tsp vanilla extract or powder

4–6 drops of liquid stevia, to sweeten (optional)

This cosy and comforting baked crumble is a firm family favourite of mine and the perfect dessert to enjoy with Sunday lunch or any special occasion. It's so simple to make and bursting with spices and flavour, and the cool, creamy vanilla whip makes it an extra special pudding.

1   Preheat the oven to 180°C. Lightly grease a 23cm x 33cm baking dish with coconut oil.

2   In a large mixing bowl, toss together the slices of apple and pear with the coconut sugar, lemon juice, cinnamon, water, starch, ginger, if using, and nutmeg. Transfer to the prepared baking dish.

3   In the same mixing bowl, add all the crumble topping ingredients and mix together well. Taste and adjust the amount of sugar or spices, as needed. Pour the topping across the apple and pear mixture in an even layer.

4   Bake in the oven for 45–50 minutes, until the topping is golden brown and the filling is bubbling at the edges. Remove from the heat and set aside to cool.

5   Meanwhile, to make the vanilla whip, carefully open the tins of chilled coconut milk without shaking them. The coconut cream should have set in a thick layer at the top of the tin. Use a spoon to scoop the cream into a mixing bowl, leaving the coconut water behind. Add the vanilla and liquid stevia, if using, and use a hand-held whisk to whisk the coconut cream for 2–3 minutes, until light and fluffy.

6   Serve the warm crumble with a dollop of vanilla whip. Any leftovers can be stored in an airtight container in the fridge for two or three days.

ANTIOXIDANT-RICH   ENERGY-BOOSTING   GOOD MOOD   SLEEP-ENHANCING

Squidgy Banoffee Pie

SERVES 6 | PER SERVING: 459 CALORIES | 10.3G PROTEIN | 63.5G CARBS | 21.6G FAT

FOR THE BASE:

80g gluten-free rolled oats

150g pitted dates, soaked in hot water for 20 minutes to soften

145g raw unsalted almonds

1 tbsp coconut flour

2 tsp vanilla extract or powder

1 tsp ground cinnamon

FOR THE CARAMEL LAYER:

150g pitted dates, soaked in hot water for 20 minutes to soften

2 tbsp raw unsalted almond butter

2 tbsp pure maple syrup

2 tsp vanilla extract or powder

1 tsp fresh lemon juice

1 large or 2 small ripe bananas, sliced

FOR THE TOP LAYER:

2 x 400ml tins of full-fat coconut milk, chilled overnight in the fridge

2 tsp vanilla extract or powder

pinch of raw cacao powder or unsweetened dark cocoa powder, to decorate

A healthier version of the traditional banoffee pie and free from gluten, dairy and refined sugar, but just as creamy, gooey and delicious. A definite people pleaser, it's sure to be a hit with everybody at special celebrations. I love to make this pie for summer parties with family and friends, and there's never anything left to bring home again.

1   First make the base. Pour the oats in a food processor or blender and blend for up to 60 seconds, until a fine flour forms. Place the oat flour and the remaining base ingredients in a food processor fitted with the regular S blade and blend until a sticky dough forms. You may want to create a coarse meal or to leave a bit more texture. Press the dough into a 12cm silicone or springform tin, or into three small tins, as pictured, and place in the freezer to set for 20 minutes.

2   To make the middle caramel layer, drain the soaked dates and blend all the ingredients except the banana together in a blender or food processor until it becomes a smooth, thick caramel sauce. Use a little water to help it blend if necessary. Smooth the caramel layer on top of the base, then layer the banana slices on top. (Save some bananas to decorate the very top of the pie.) Place the pie back in the freezer to set.

3   To make the top cream layer, carefully open up the chilled tins of coconut milk without shaking them. The cream should have separated from the liquid. Spoon out the cream and place it in a mixing bowl. Add the vanilla and use a hand-held electric whisk or a fork to briskly whisk the cream until it's frothy. Smooth the cream layer on top of the pie, ensuring it's even.

4   Add the remaining banana slices and finish with a sprinkle of cacao powder to decorate. Serve chilled. The banoffee pie can be stored in the fridge in an airtight container for two or three days.

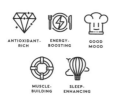

ANTIOXIDANT-RICH   ENERGY-BOOSTING   GOOD MOOD

MUSCLE-BUILDING   SLEEP-ENHANCING

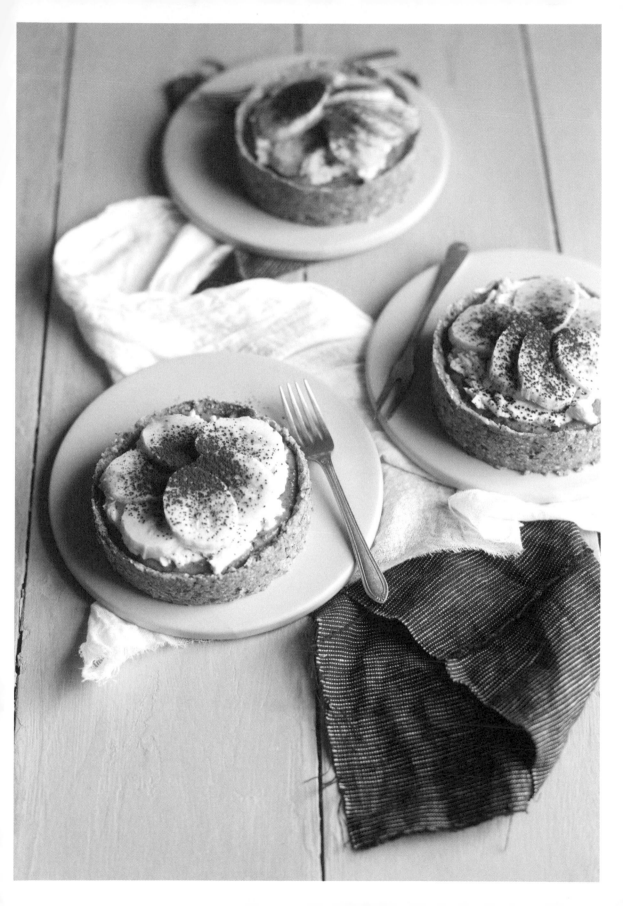

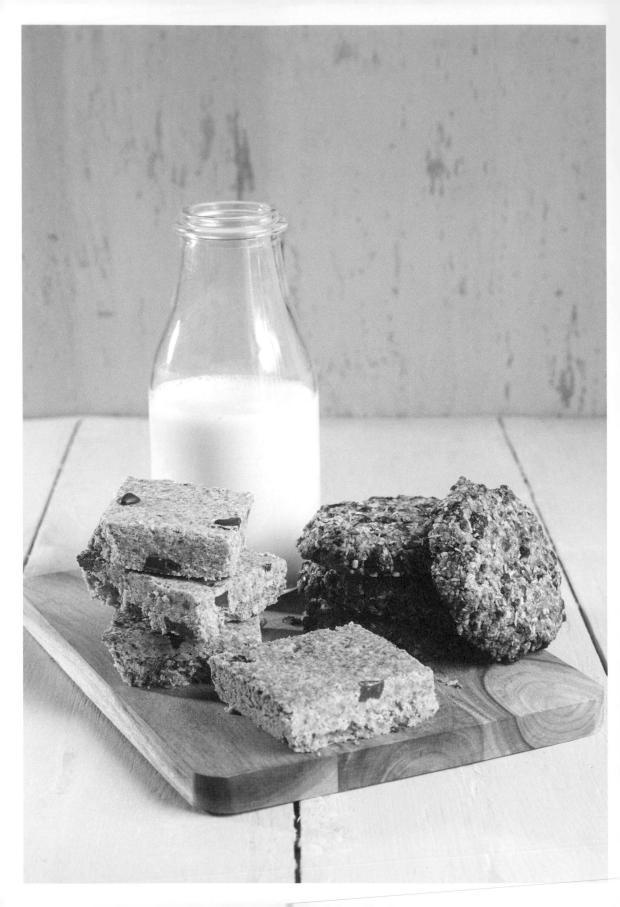

Chocolate Chip Cookie Dough Brownies

MAKES 8 BROWNIES | PER BROWNIE: 288 CALORIES | 5.8G PROTEIN | 37.8G CARBS | 13.1G FAT

160g gluten-free rolled oats

115g brown rice flour

½ tsp gluten-free baking powder

110g pitted dates, soaked in hot water for 20 minutes to soften

3 tbsp coconut oil, melted, plus extra to grease

3 tbsp raw unsalted almond butter

3 tbsp coconut sugar

1 tsp vanilla extract

50g dark chocolate (at least 80–90% cocoa content), broken into small pieces

ANTIOXIDANT-RICH   ENERGY-BOOSTING

GOOD MOOD   MUSCLE-BUILDING

If you're finding it difficult to choose between a chocolate chip cookie or a fudge brownie for your special sweet treat, then you have come to the right place. These brownies are the perfect combination of a chocolate chip cookie and a gooey fudge brownie, made with healthier ingredients and naturally sweetened with coconut sugar and dates. Decision made!

1   Preheat the oven to 190°C. Lightly grease a medium-sized baking tray with coconut oil or line with non-stick baking paper.

2   Place the oats in a blender and blend for 60 seconds, until a fine flour forms. Tip the oats into a large mixing bowl with the brown rice flour and baking powder and mix together.

3   Drain the dates and place them in a blender or food processor with the melted coconut oil, almond butter, coconut sugar and vanilla extract. Blend until a smooth caramel forms. Mix the caramel into the dry ingredients until a thick dough forms. Gently fold in the chocolate pieces, ensuring it's mixed in evenly.

4   Press the dough into the tray in an even layer. Bake in the oven for 12–15 minutes, until firm to touch and turning golden brown. Allow to cool for 10 minutes before slicing into squares and serving. The brownies can be stored in an airtight container in a cool, dry place for up to three days.

Raspberry Coconut Ice Cream Brownie Bars

MAKES 6 BARS | PER SERVING: 272 CALORIES | 5G PROTEIN | 24.8G CARBS | 19.3G FAT

80g raw unsalted almonds

75g raw pecans

35g raw cacao powder

130g dates, pitted and soaked in hot water for 20 minutes to soften

1 tsp vanilla extract

2½ tbsp coconut oil, melted

FOR THE RASPBERRY COCONUT ICE CREAM:

1 x 400ml tin of full-fat coconut milk, chilled overnight in the fridge

60g fresh raspberries

3 tbsp coconut oil, melted

1 tbsp pure maple syrup or honey

2 tsp vanilla extract or powder

ANTIOXIDANT-
RICH   ENERGY-
BOOSTING

GOOD
MOOD

Love ice cream? Love brownies? Two of my all-time favourite desserts are combined here in these delicious ice cream brownie bars. They make the best sweet treat on a warm day and they're fun to eat too. Finger food at its finest.

1   Place the almonds, pecans and cacao powder in a food processor and blend until a crumbly mixture forms. Transfer to a mixing bowl.

2   Place the soaked and drained dates and vanilla in the food processor and blend until smooth. Stop to scrape down the sides and use a splash of warm water to help it blend if necessary. Add the nut and cacao mixture and the melted coconut oil and pulse to combine until the mixture forms a thick, clumpy dough.

3   Line two loaf tins with non-stick baking paper. Divide the brownie mixture in half and pack the base of each tin with half of the mixture. Press down firmly to form a thin, even layer. Place the tins in the freezer to set for 20–30 minutes.

4   To make the ice cream, carefully open the tin of chilled coconut cream without shaking it. The thick coconut cream should have separated from the water. Spoon the coconut cream into a blender or food processor. Add the raspberries, melted coconut oil, maple syrup and vanilla to the coconut cream and blend on high until a smooth ice cream forms.

5   Remove the two brownie tins from the freezer. Spoon the ice cream on top of one of the brownie layers, smoothing it across the top with a spatula. Carefully lift the second layer of brownie out of the tin, peel off the paper and place the brownie on top of the ice cream layer, pressing down very gently.

6   Place it back in the freezer to set for 20 minutes, then remove and slice into bars using a sharp knife. Serve chilled. Any leftovers can be stored in an airtight container in the fridge for two days, but the bars are best eaten on the day that they're made.

Maple and Cinnamon Blondies

MAKES 9 BLONDIES | PER BLONDIE: 254 CALORIES | 6G PROTEIN | 30G CARBS | 12G FAT

coconut oil, to grease

1 x 400g tin of chickpeas, drained and rinsed

235g pure maple syrup or honey

130g smooth unsalted almond butter or peanut butter

2 tsp vanilla extract or powder

1 tsp ground cinnamon

1 tsp gluten-free baking powder

100g dark chocolate (70–85% cacao), chopped into chunks, or 50g pecan halves (optional)

These flourless and oil-free blondies use chickpeas as the secret healthy and protein-rich ingredient. They're gluten free, naturally sweetened and a delicious way to sneak some extra fibre-rich beans into your diet. I love them with a cup of tea as a treat-day snack after a workout.

1   Preheat the oven to 190°C. Lightly grease a 23cm square baking tin with coconut oil or line with non-stick baking paper.

2   Place the chickpeas, maple syrup, almond butter, vanilla, cinnamon and baking powder in a food processor and blend on high for 3–5 minutes, scraping down the sides as needed, until the mixture is smooth and well blended. Stir in the dark chocolate chunks or pecan halves, if using.

3   Pour the mixture into the prepared baking tin and bake in the oven for 35–40 minutes, until golden brown with crisp, firm edges. Don't worry if the centre is still soft to touch, as it will gently firm up as they cool. Let the blondies cool before slicing and serving. Store them in an airtight container in the fridge for three or four days.

Index